The Morphy Richards Slow Cooker Cookbook

Samuel Joyce

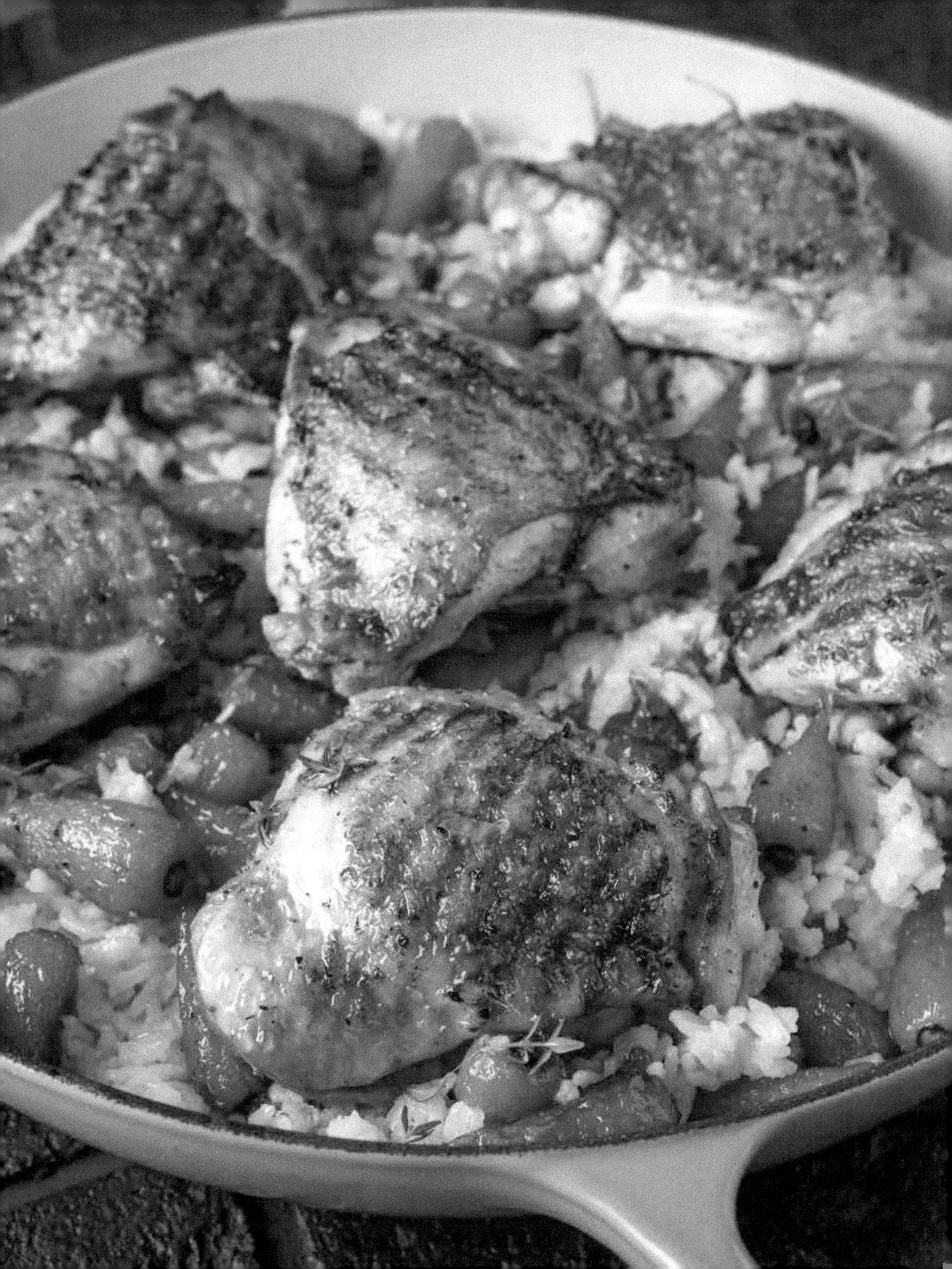

CONTENTS

FISH & SEAFOOD RECIPES 84

INTRODUCTION

10 top tips for using a slow cooker

Slow cookers are cheap to buy, economical to use and they're great for making the most of budget ingredients. They offer a healthier, low-fat method of cooking and require the minimum amount of effort. Really, what's not to love?

1. Cut down your prep time

One of the main attractions for many people is the ease of a slow cooker, so when you're looking for recipes, avoid those that suggest a lot of pre-preparation. For many dishes, particularly soups and stews, you really can just throw all the ingredients in. It can be nice to cook the onions beforehand, as the flavour is different to when you put them in raw, but experiment both ways as you may find you prefer one. It can also be good to brown meat to give it some colour, but again, this is not essential.

2. Prepare for slow cooking the night before

If you're short on time in the morning, prepare everything you need for your slow-cooked meal the night before, put it into the slow-cooker dish, cover and store in the fridge overnight. Ideally the dish should be as close to room temperature as possible, so get it out of the fridge when you wake up and leave it for 20 minutes before turning the cooker on. If you need to heat your dish beforehand, then put the ingredients in a different container and transfer them in the morning.

3. Choose cheap cuts

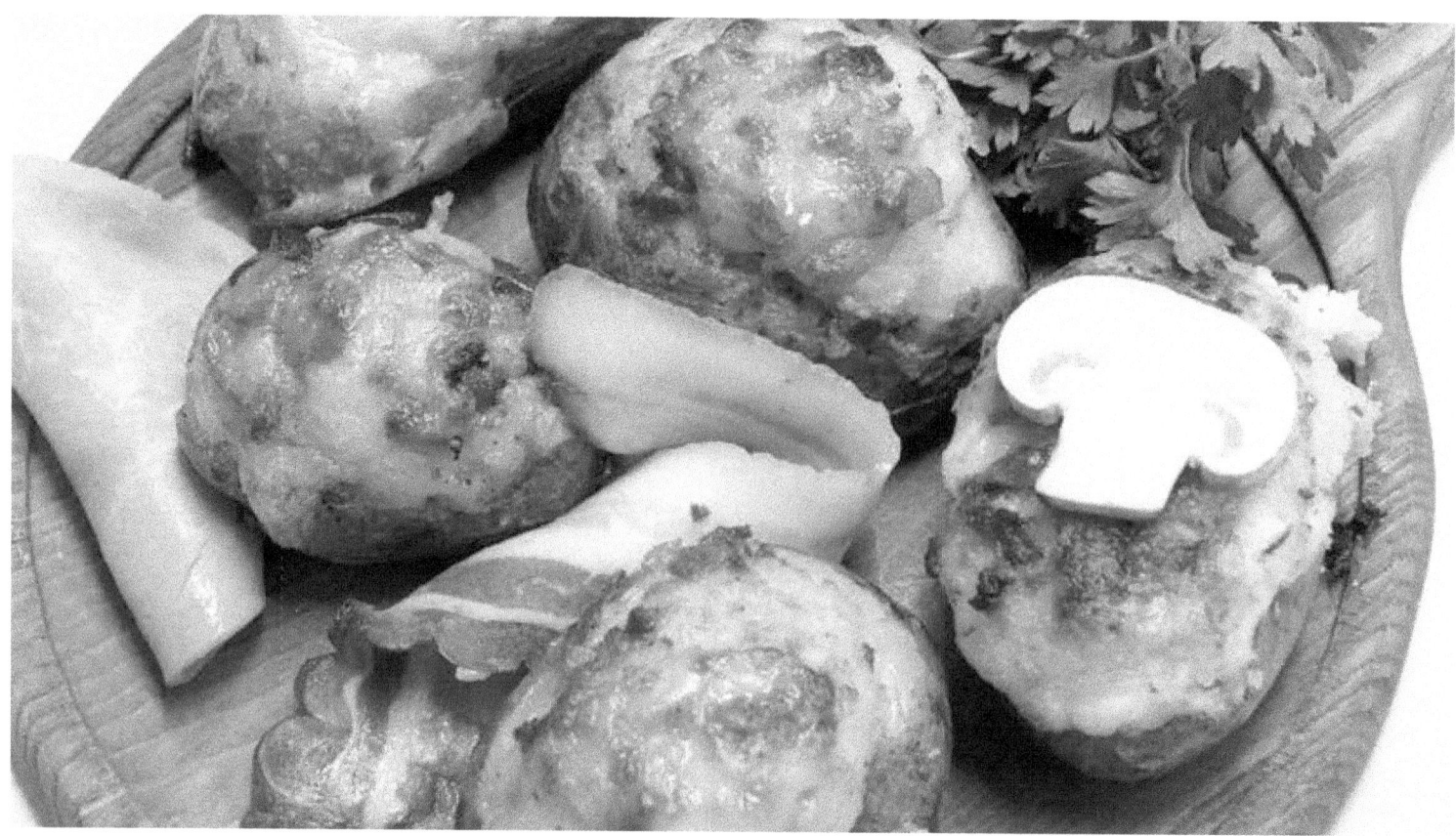

Slow cookers are great for cooking cheaper cuts like beef brisket, pork shoulder, lamb shoulder and chicken thighs. You can also use less meat, as slow cooking really extracts a meaty flavour that permeates the whole dish. Bulk up with vegetables instead.

4. Trim fat from meat before slow cooking

You don't need to add oil to a slow cooker – the contents won't catch as long as there's enough moisture in there. You don't need a lot of fat on your meat either. Normally when you fry meat, a lot of the fat drains away, but this won't happen in a slow cooker so trim it off – otherwise you might find you have pools of oil in your stew. Removing the fat will give you a healthier result, and it'll still be tasty.

5. Reduce liquid when using a slow cooker

Because your slow cooker will have a tightly sealed lid, the liquid won't evaporate so if you're adapting a standard recipe, it's best to reduce the liquid by roughly a third. It should just cover the meat and vegetables. Don't overfill your slow cooker, or it may start leaking out the top, and the food won't cook so well. Half to two-thirds full is ideal – certainly no more than three-quarters.

6. Use flour to thicken sauces

Just as the the liquid doesn't reduce, it also doesn't thicken. You can roll meat in a small amount of seasoned flour before adding it to the slow cooker or use a little cornflour at the end. If you want to do the latter, take a teaspoon or two of cornflour and mix it to a paste with a little cold water. Stir into your simmering slow cooker contents, then

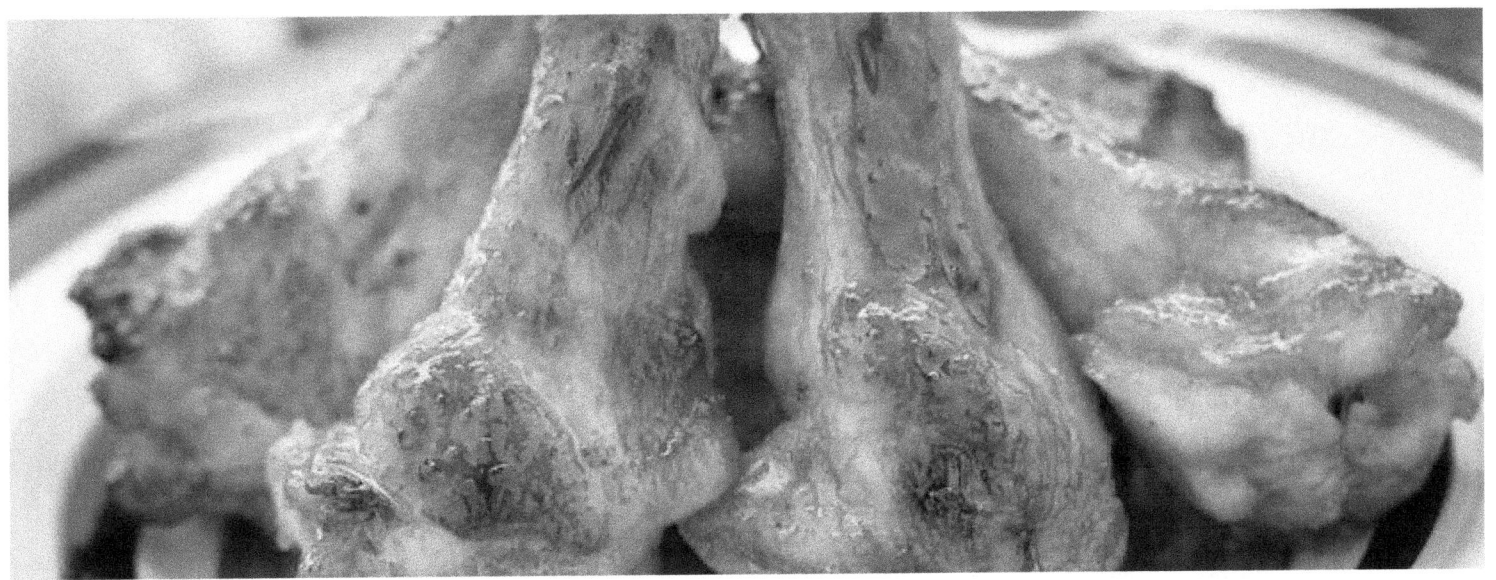

replace the lid.

7. Use the slow cooker low setting

Ginny has been working with slow-cookers for over a decade, and her advice is to use the 'Low' setting as much as you can, finding that most dishes really benefit from a slow, gentle heat to really bring out the flavours. This also means you won't need to worry if you're heading out for the day – it'll take care of itself. "I think of it as my cook fairy making my dinner while I'm out," says Ginny.

8. Leave your slow cooker recipe alone

Slow cookers are designed to do their own thing, so you don't need to keep checking the contents. Every time you take the lid off it will release some of the heat, so if you keep doing this you'll have to increase the cooking time.

9. Add all ingredients at the start (most of the time)

Ideally you want to choose recipes where most, if not all, of the ingredients can be added at the beginning, leaving you free to do other things. However, in most cases, pasta, rice and fresh herbs will need to be added towards the end.

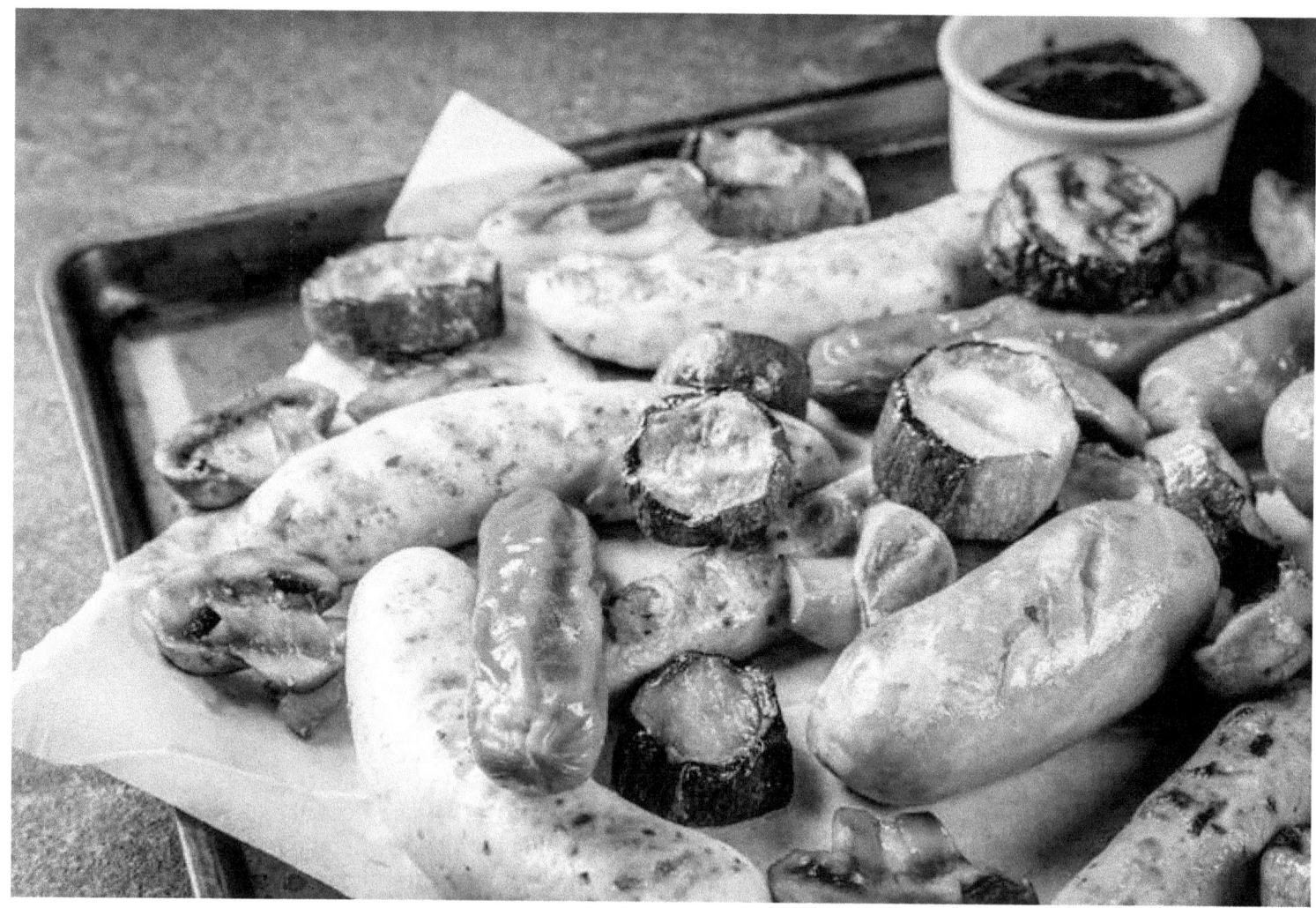

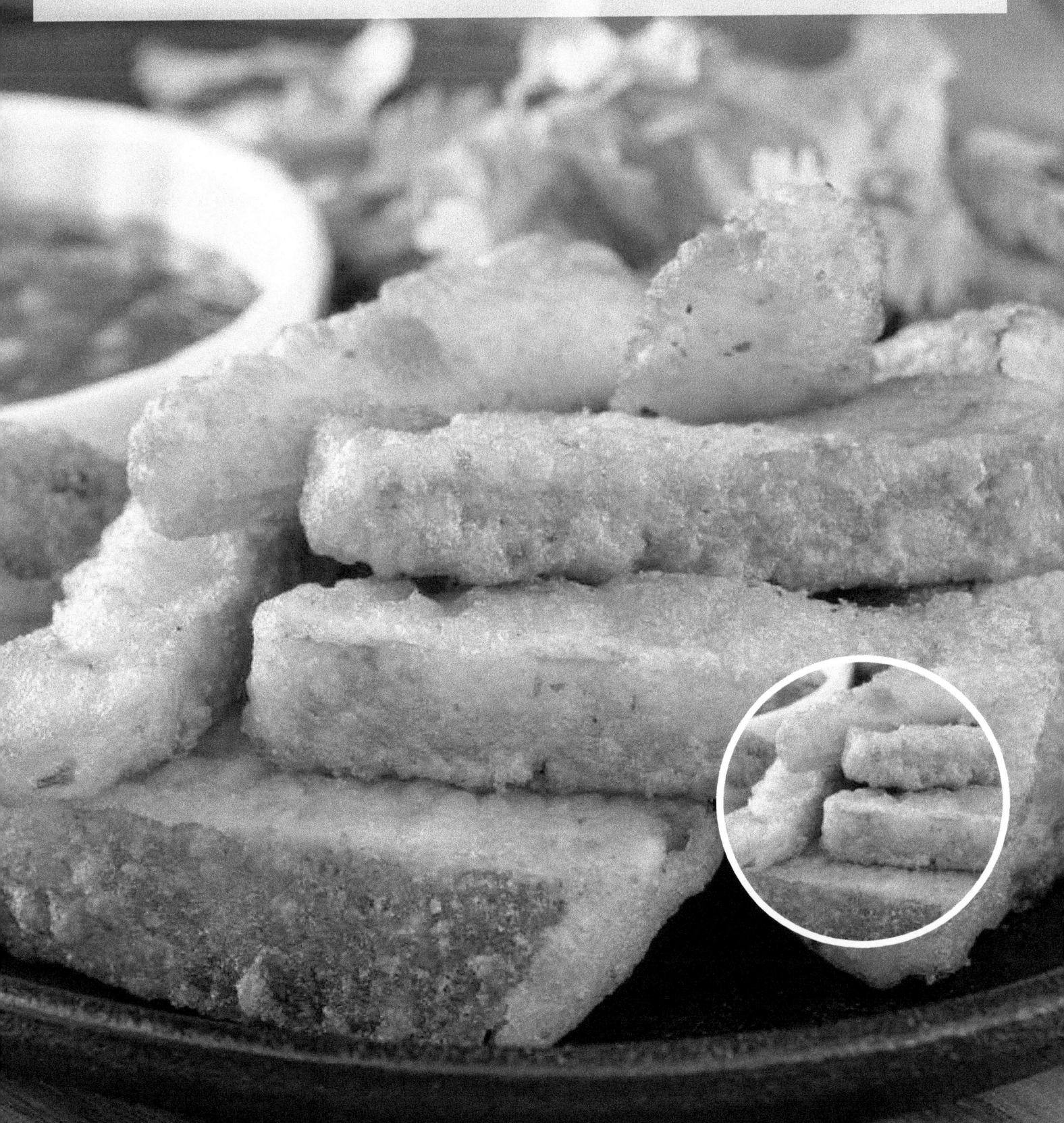

APPETIZERS RECIPES

Artichoke Bread Pudding

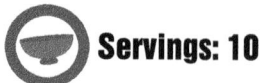 **Servings: 10**   **Cooking Time: 6 1/2 hours**

Ingredients:

- 6 cups bread cubes
- 6 artichoke hearts, drained and chopped
- 1/2 cup grated Parmesan
- 4 eggs
- 1/2 cup sour cream
- 1 cup milk
- 4 oz. spinach, chopped
- 1 tablespoon chopped parsley
- 2 tablespoons olive oil
- Salt and pepper to taste
- 1/2 teaspoon dried oregano
- 1/2 teaspoon dried basil

Directions:

1. Combine the bread cubes, artichoke hearts and Parmesan in your Crock Pot. Add the spinach and parsley as well.
2. In a bowl, mix the eggs, sour cream, milk, oregano and basil, as well as salt and pepper.
3. Pour this mixture over the bread and press the bread slightly to make sure it soaks up all the liquid.
4. Cover the pot with its lid and cook on low settings for 6 hours.
5. The bread can be served both warm and chilled.

Artichoke Dip

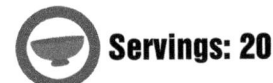 **Servings: 20**   **Cooking Time: 6 1/4 hours**

Ingredients:

- 2 sweet onions, chopped
- 1 red chili, chopped
- 2 garlic cloves, chopped
- 1 jar artichoke hearts, drained and chopped
- 1 cup cream cheese
- 1 cup heavy cream
- 2 oz. blue cheese, crumbled
- 2 tablespoons chopped cilantro

Directions:

1. Mix the onions, chili, garlic, artichoke hearts, cream cheese, heavy cream and blue cheese in a Crock Pot.
2. Cook on low settings for 6 hours.
3. When done, stir in the cilantro and serve the dip warm or chilled.

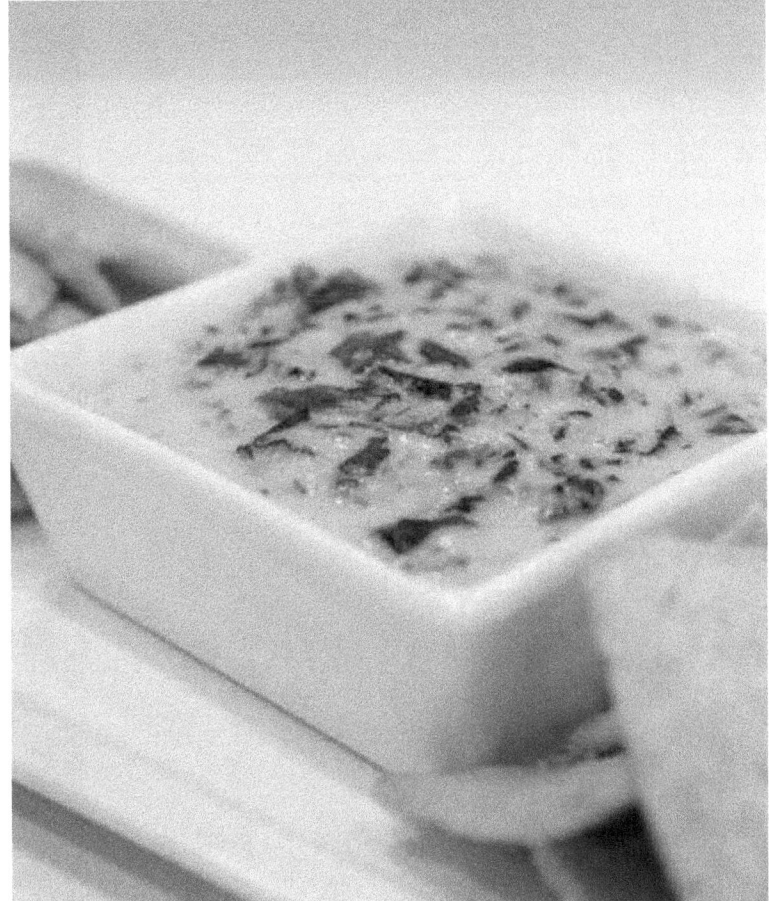

Asian Marinated Mushrooms

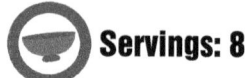 Servings: 8   Cooking Time: 8 1/4 hours

Ingredients:

- 2 pounds mushrooms
- 1 cup soy sauce
- 1 cup water
- 1/2 cup brown sugar
- 1/4 cup rice vinegar
- 1/2 teaspoon chili powder

Directions:

1. Combine all the ingredients in your Crock Pot.
2. Cover the crock pot and cook on low settings for 8 hours.
3. Allow to cool in the pot before serving.

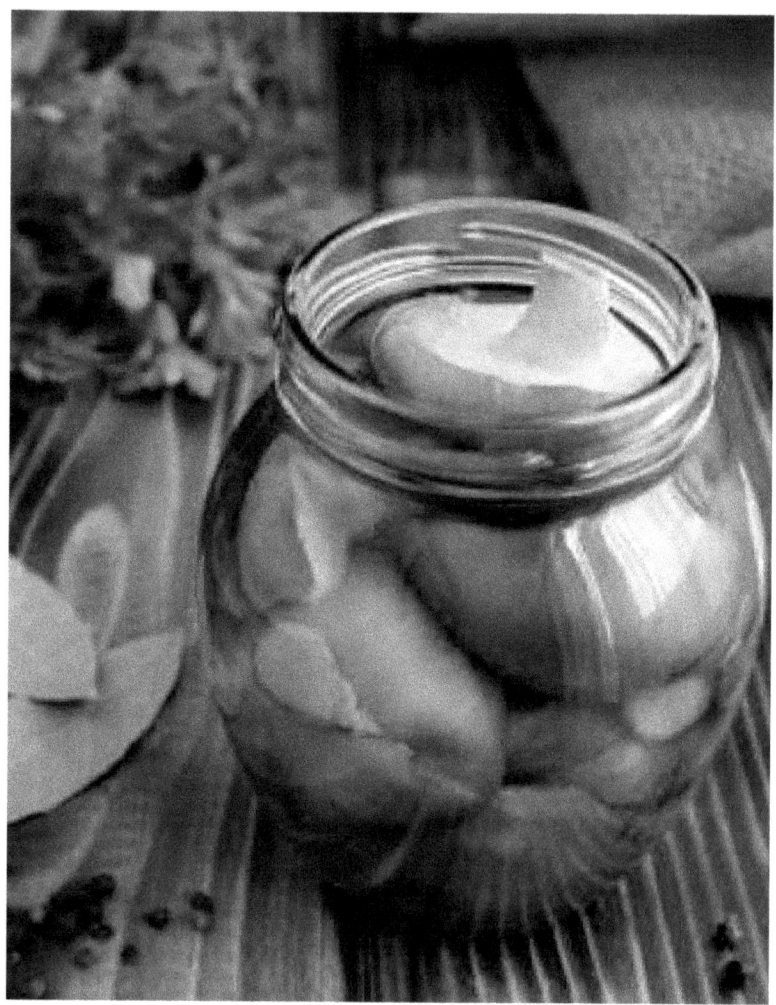

Blue Cheese Chicken Wings

 **Servings: 8**   **Cooking Time: 7 1/4 hours**

Ingredients:

- 4 pounds chicken wings
- 1/2 cup buffalo sauce
- 1/2 cup spicy tomato sauce
- 1 tablespoon tomato paste
- 2 tablespoons apple cider vinegar
- 1 tablespoon Worcestershire sauce
- 1 cup sour cream
- 2 oz. blue cheese, crumbled
- 1 thyme sprig

Directions:

1. Combine the buffalo sauce, tomato sauce, vinegar, Worcestershire sauce, sour cream, blue cheese and thyme in a Crock Pot.
2. Add the chicken wings and toss them until evenly coated.
3. Cook on low settings for 7 hours.
4. Serve the chicken wings preferably warm.

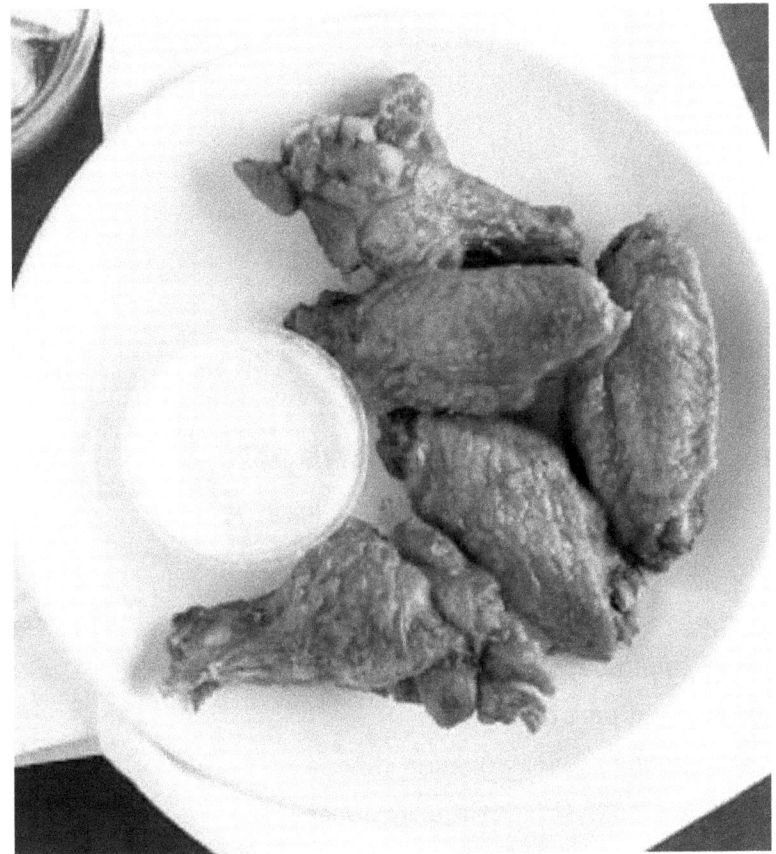

Bacon Chicken Sliders

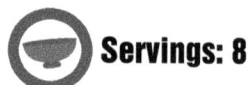 **Servings: 8**   **Cooking Time: 4 1/2 hours**

Ingredients:

- 2 pounds ground chicken
- 1 egg
- 1/2 cup breadcrumbs
- 1 shallot, chopped
- Salt and pepper to taste
- 8 bacon slices

Directions:

1. Mix the chicken, egg, breadcrumbs and shallot in a bowl. Add salt and pepper to taste and give it a good mix.
2. Form small sliders then wrap each slider in a bacon slice.
3. Place the sliders in a Crock Pot.
4. Cover with its lid and cook on high settings for 4 hours, making sure to flip them over once during cooking.
5. Serve them warm.

Bacon Crab Dip

 Servings: 20   **Cooking Time: 2 1/4 hours**

Ingredients:

- 1 pound bacon, diced
- 1 cup cream cheese
- 1/2 cup grated Parmesan cheese
- 1 teaspoon Worcestershire sauce
- 1 teaspoon Dijon mustard
- 1 can crab meat, drained and shredded
- 1 teaspoon hot sauce

Directions:

1. Heat a skillet over medium flame and add the bacon. Sauté for 5 minutes until fat begins to drain out.
2. Transfer the bacon in a Crock Pot.
3. Stir in the remaining ingredients and cook on high settings for 2 hours.
4. Serve the dip warm or chilled.

Bacon Baked Potatoes

 Servings: 8   Cooking Time: 3 1/4 hours

Ingredients:

- 3 pounds new potatoes, halved
- 8 slices bacon, chopped
- 1 teaspoon dried rosemary
- 1/4 cup chicken stock
- Salt and pepper to taste

Directions:

1. Heat a skillet over medium flame and stir in the bacon. Cook until crisp.
2. Place the potatoes in a Crock Pot. Add the bacon bits and its fat, as well as rosemary, salt and pepper and mix until evenly distributed.
3. Pour in the stock and cook on high heat for 3 hours.
4. Serve the potatoes warm.

Beer Cheese Fondue

 Servings: 8   Cooking Time: 2 1/4 hours

Ingredients:

- 1 shallot, chopped
- 1 garlic clove, minced
- 1 cup grated Gruyere cheese
- 2 cups grated Cheddar
- 1 tablespoon cornstarch
- 1 teaspoon Dijon mustard
- 1/2 teaspoon cumin seeds
- 1 cup beer
- Salt and pepper to taste

Directions:

1. Combine the shallot, garlic, cheeses, cornstarch, mustard, cumin seeds and beer in your Crock Pot.
2. Add salt and pepper to taste and mix well.
3. Cover the pot with its lid and cook on high settings for 2 hours.
4. Serve the fondue warm.

Beer BBQ Meatballs

 **Servings: 10**   **Cooking Time: 7 1/2 hours**

Ingredients:

- 2 pounds ground pork
- 1 pound ground beef
- 1 carrot, grated
- 2 shallots, chopped
- 1 egg
- 1/2 cup breadcrumbs
- 1/2 teaspoon cumin powder
- Salt and pepper to taste
- 1 cup dark beer
- 1 cup BBQ sauce
- 1 bay leaf
- 1/2 teaspoon chili powder
- 1 teaspoon apple cider vinegar

Directions:

1. Mix the ground pork and beef in a bowl. Add the carrot, shallots, egg, breadcrumbs, cumin, salt and pepper and mix well. Form small meatballs and place them on your chopping board.
2. For the beer sauce, combine the beer, BBQ sauce, bay leaf, chili powder and vinegar in a Crock Pot.
3. Place the meatballs in the pot and cover with its lid.
4. Cook on low settings for 7 hours.
5. Serve the meatballs warm or chilled.

Boiled Peanuts with Skin On

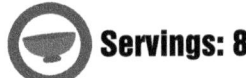 **Servings: 8**　　 **Cooking Time: 7 1/4 hours**

Ingredients:

- 2 pounds uncooked, whole peanuts
- 1/2 cup salt
- 4 cups water

Directions:

1. Combine all the ingredients in your Crock Pot.
2. Cover and cook on low settings for 7 hours.
3. Drain and allow to cool down before servings.

Bean Queso

 Servings: 10　　 **Cooking Time: 6 1/4 hours**

Ingredients:

- 1 can black beans, drained
- 1 cup chopped green chiles
- 1/2 cup red salsa
- 1 teaspoon dried oregano
- 1/2 teaspoon cumin powder
- 1 cup light beer
- 1 1/2 cups grated Cheddar
- Salt and pepper to taste

Directions:

1. Combine the beans, chiles, oregano, cumin, salsa, beer and cheese in your Crock Pot.
2. Add salt and pepper as needed and cook on low settings for 6 hours.
3. Serve the bean queso warm.

Balsamico Pulled Pork

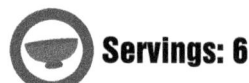 Servings: 6 Cooking Time: 8 1/4 hours

Ingredients:

- 2 pounds boneless pork shoulder
- 2 tablespoons honey
- 1/4 cup balsamic vinegar
- 1/4 cup hoisin sauce
- 1 tablespoon Dijon mustard
- 1/4 cup chicken stock
- 2 garlic cloves, minced
- 2 shallots, sliced
- 2 tablespoons soy sauce

Directions:

1. Combine the honey, vinegar, hoisin sauce, mustard, stock, garlic, shallots and soy sauce in your Crock Pot.
2. Add the pork shoulder and roll it in the mixture until evenly coated.
3. Cover the Crock Pot and cook on low settings for 8 hours.
4. When done, shred the meat into fine pieces and serve warm or chilled.

Bourbon Glazed Sausages

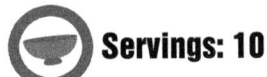 **Servings: 10** **Cooking Time: 4 1/4 hours**

Ingredients:

- 3 pounds small sausage links
- 1/2 cup apricot preserves
- 1/4 cup maple syrup
- 2 tablespoons Bourbon

Directions:

1. Combine all the ingredients in your Crock Pot.
2. Cover with its lid and cook on low settings for 4 hours.
3. Serve the glazed sausages warm or chilled, preferably with cocktail sticks.

Bacon Wrapped Chicken Livers

 Servings: 6 **Cooking Time: 3 1/2 hours**

Ingredients:

- 2 pounds chicken livers
- Bacon slices as needed

Directions:

1. Wrap each chicken liver in one slice of bacon and place all the livers in your crock pot.
2. Cook on high heat for 3 hours.
3. Serve warm or chilled.

Bacon Wrapped Dates

 **Servings: 8**   **Cooking Time: 1 3/4 hours**

Ingredients:

- 16 dates, pitted
- 16 almonds
- 16 slices bacon

Directions:

1. Stuff each date with an almond.
2. Wrap each date in bacon and place the wrapped dates in your Crock Pot.
3. Cover with its lid and cook on high settings for 1 1/4 hours.
4. Serve warm or chilled.

Bacon New Potatoes

 Servings: 6   **Cooking Time: 3 1/4 hours**

Ingredients:

- 3 pounds new potatoes, washed and halved
- 12 slices bacon, chopped
- 2 tablespoons white wine
- Salt and pepper to taste
- 1 rosemary sprig

Directions:

1. Place the potatoes, wine and rosemary in your Crock Pot.
2. Add salt and pepper to taste and top with chopped bacon.
3. Cook on high settings for 3 hours.
4. Serve the potatoes warm.

Bacon Black Bean Dip

 **Servings: 6**   **Cooking Time: 6 1/4 hours**

Ingredients:

- 6 bacon slices
- 2 cans black beans, drained
- 2 shallots, sliced
- 1 garlic cloves, chopped
- 1 cup red salsa
- 1/2 cup beef stock
- 1 tablespoon brown sugar
- 1 tablespoon molasses
- 1/2 teaspoon chili powder
- 1 tablespoon apple cider vinegar
- 2 tablespoons Bourbon
- Salt and pepper to taste

Directions:

1. Heat a skillet over medium flame and add the bacon. Cook until crisp then transfer the bacon and its fat in your Crock Pot.
2. Stir in the remaining ingredients and cook on low settings for 6 hours.
3. When done, partially mash the beans and serve the dip right away.

Baba Ganoush

 **Servings: 4**   **Cooking Time: 4 1/4 hours**

Ingredients:

- 1 large eggplant, halved
- 2 garlic cloves, minced
- 2 tablespoons olive oil
- 1 tablespoon tahini paste
- 1 tablespoon lemon juice
- 1 tablespoon chopped parsley
- Salt and pepper to taste

Directions:

1. Spread the garlic over each half of eggplant. Season them with salt and pepper and drizzle with olive oil.
2. Place the eggplant halves in your Crock Pot and cook on low settings for 4 hours.
3. When done, scoop out the eggplant flesh and place it in a bowl. Mash it with a fork.
4. Stir in the tahini paste, lemon juice and parsley and mix well.
5. Serve the dip fresh.

Candied Kielbasa

 Servings: 8   **Cooking Time: 6 1/4 hours**

Ingredients:

- 2 pounds kielbasa sausages
- 1/2 cup brown sugar
- 1 cup BBQ sauce
- 1 teaspoon prepared horseradish
- 1/2 teaspoon black pepper
- 1/4 teaspoon cumin powder

Directions:

1. Combine all the ingredients in a Crock Pot, adding salt if needed.
2. Cook on low settings for 6 hours.
3. Serve the kielbasa warm or chilled.

Caramelized Onion and Cranberry Dip

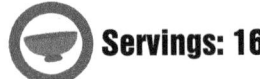 **Servings: 16**   **Cooking Time: 6 1/4 hours**

Ingredients:

- 2 tablespoons olive oil
- 4 red onions, sliced
- 1 apple, peeled and diced
- 1 cup frozen cranberries
- 1/4 cup balsamic vinegar
- 1/4 cup fresh orange juice
- 2 tablespoons brown sugar
- 1 teaspoon orange zest
- 1 bay leaf
- 1 thyme sprig
- 1 teaspoon salt

Directions:

1. Heat the oil in a skillet and stir in the onions. Cook for 10 minutes until the onions begin to caramelize.
2. Transfer the onions in a Crock Pot and stir in the remaining ingredients.
3. Cover with a lid and cook on low settings for 6 hours.
4. Serve the dip chilled.

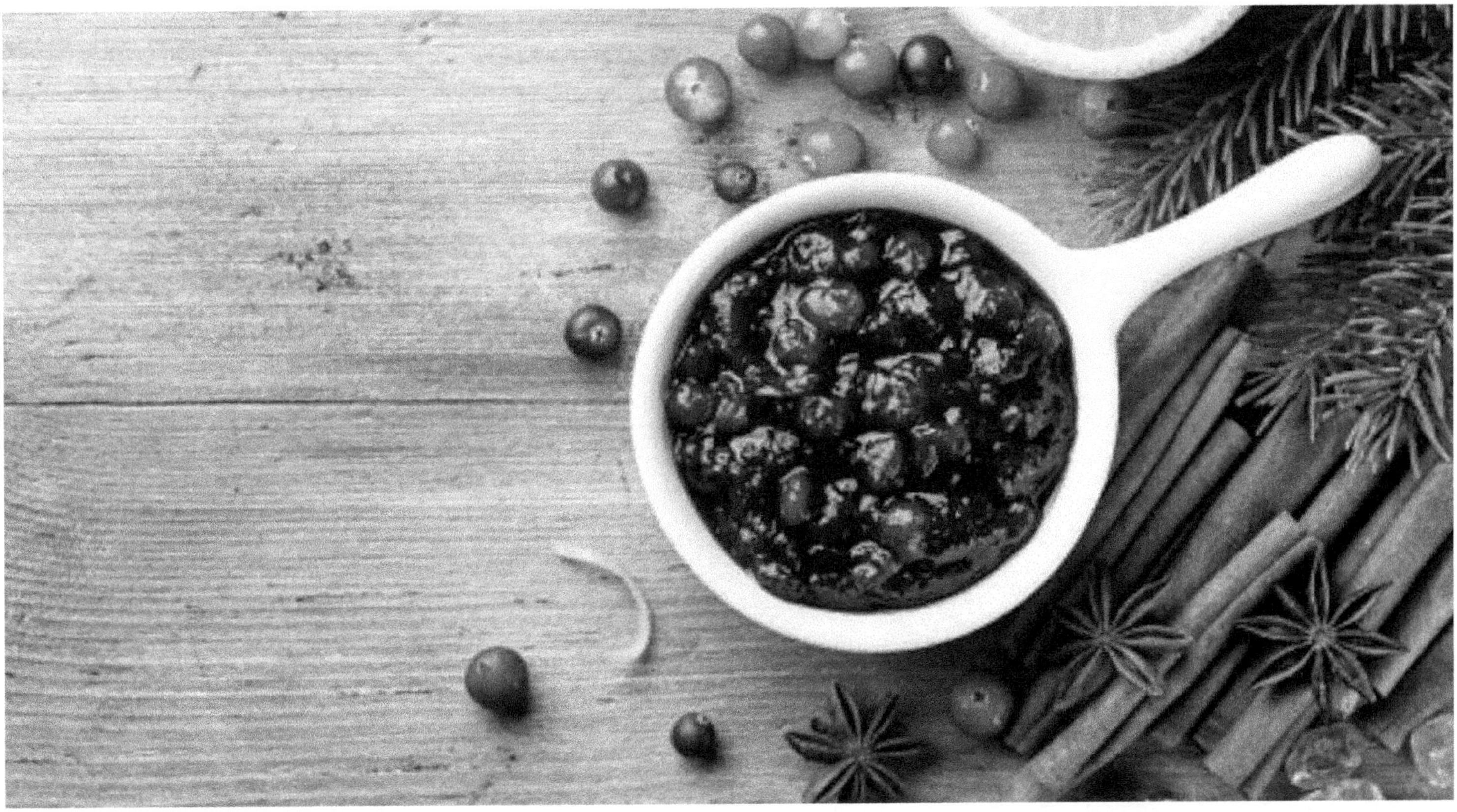

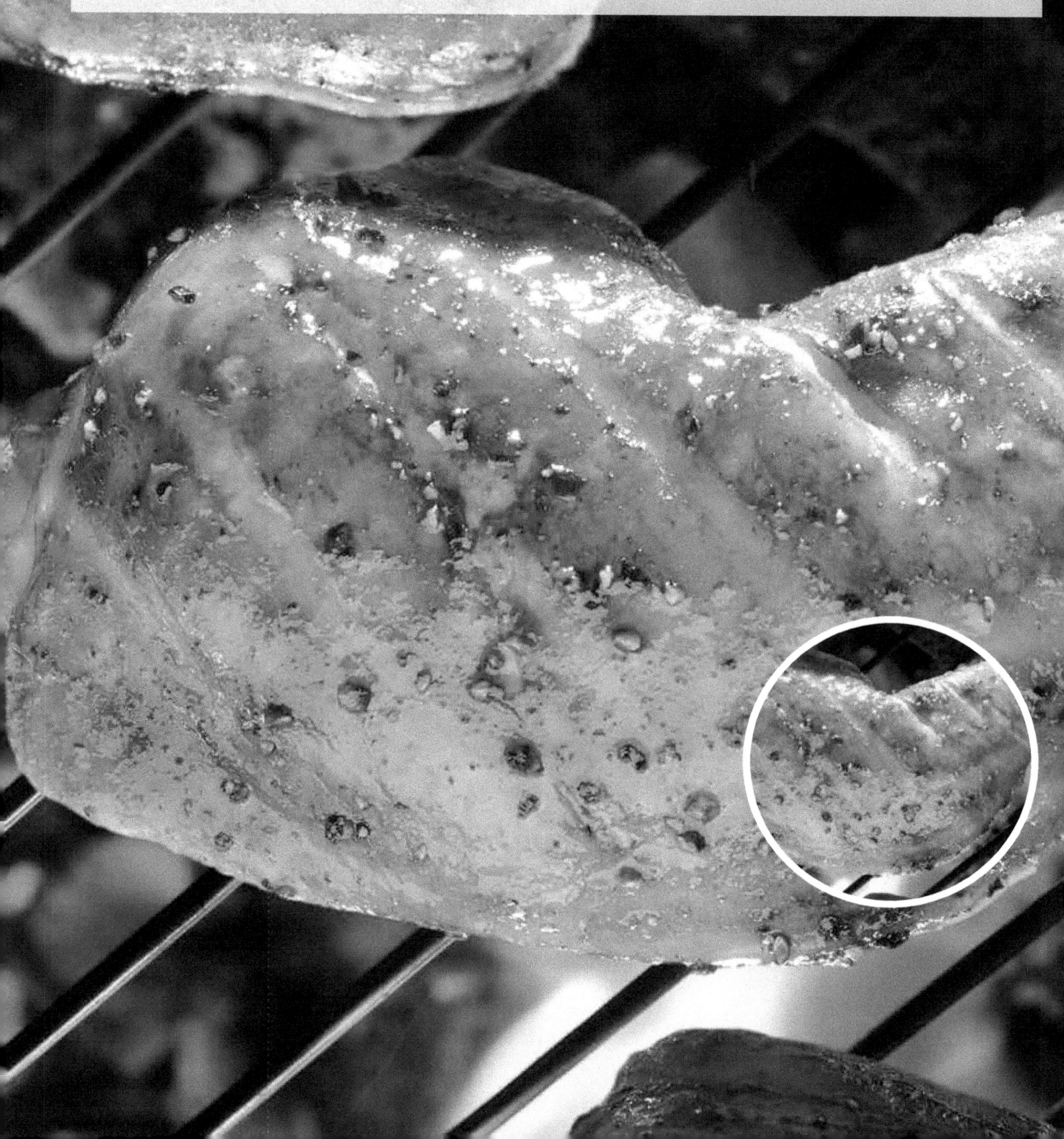

POULTRY RECIPES

Bacon Chicken

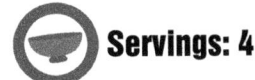 **Servings: 4**　　 **Cooking Time: 7 hours**

Ingredients:

- 4 bacon slices, cooked
- 4 chicken drumsticks
- ½ cup of water
- ¼ tomato juice
- 1 teaspoon salt
- ½ teaspoon ground black pepper

Directions:

1. Sprinkle the chicken drumsticks with the salt and ground black pepper.
2. Then wrap every chicken drumstick in the bacon and arrange it in the Crock Pot.
3. Add water and tomato juice.
4. Cook the meal on Low for 7 hours.

Asian Sesame Chicken

 Servings: 12　　 **Cooking Time: 8 hours**

Ingredients:

- 12 chicken thighs, bones and skin removed
- 2 tablespoons sesame oil
- 3 tablespoons water
- 3 tablespoons soy sauce
- 1 thumb-size ginger, sliced thinly

Directions:

1. Place all ingredients in the crockpot.
2. Stir all ingredients to combine.
3. Close the lid and cook on low for 8 hours or on high for 6 hours.
4. Once cooked, garnish with toasted sesame seeds.

Balsamic Chicken

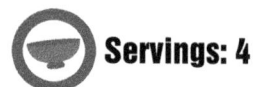 **Servings: 4**   **Cooking Time: 5 hours**

Ingredients:

- 2 cups Brussels sprouts, halved
- 4 chicken breasts, skinless and boneless
- 2 cups red potatoes, halved
- ¼ cup balsamic vinegar
- ¼ cup honey
- 1/3 cup chicken stock
- 2 tablespoons Dijon mustard
- ½ teaspoon rosemary, dried
- 1 teaspoon thyme, dried
- ½ teaspoon oregano, dried
- ½ teaspoon red pepper flakes, crushed
- 2 garlic cloves, minced
- Salt and black pepper to the taste
- 1 tablespoon parsley, chopped

Directions:

1. In your Crock Pot, mix Brussels sprouts with chicken, potatoes, vinegar, honey, stock, mustard, rosemary, thyme, oregano, pepper flakes, garlic, salt and pepper, stir, cover and cook on Low for 5 hours.
2. Add parsley, stir, divide between plates and serve.

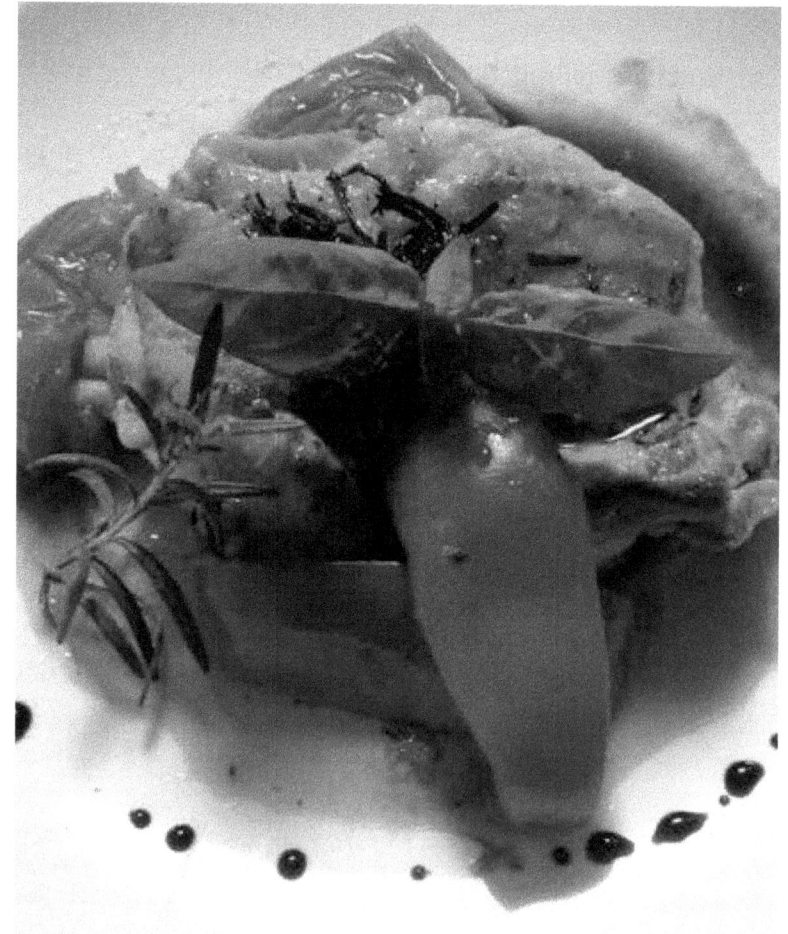

Bali Style Chicken

 **Servings: 4**   **Cooking Time: 4 hours**

Ingredients:

- 4 chicken drumsticks
- 1 teaspoon chili powder
- 1 teaspoon allspices
- 1 teaspoon minced garlic
- 2 tablespoons olive oil
- ½ cup tomato juice
- 1 jalapeno pepper, chopped

Directions:

1. Mix chili powder, allspices, minced garlic, olive oil, jalapeno pepper, and tomato juice in the bowl.
2. Add chicken drumsticks and mix the mixture. Marinate the chicken for 30 minutes.
3. Then transfer the chicken with tomato juice mixture in the Crock Pot and close the lid.
4. Cook the chicken on High for 4 hours.

Avocado Chicken Salad

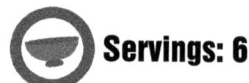 **Servings: 6**   **Cooking Time: 3.5 hours**

Ingredients:

- 1-pound chicken fillet, chopped
- 1 teaspoon salt
- 1 teaspoon ground black pepper
- ½ cup of water
- 1 avocado, pitted, peeled, chopped
- 1 tomato, chopped
- 2 tablespoons plain yogurt
- 1 tablespoon lemon juice

Directions:

1. Mix chicken fillet with salt and ground black pepper.
2. Put the chicken in the Crock Pot, add water, and cook on High for 3.5 hours.
3. Meanwhile, mix avocado with tomato in the salad bowl.
4. In the shallow bowl mix lemon juice and plain yogurt.
5. When the chicken is cooked, add it in the salad and mix well.
6. Sprinkle the meal with plain yogurt mixture.

Algerian Chicken

 **Servings: 2**   **Cooking Time: 4 hours**

Ingredients:

- 6 oz chicken breast, skinless, boneless, sliced
- 1 teaspoon peanut oil
- 1 teaspoon harissa
- 1 teaspoon tomato paste
- 1 tablespoon sesame oil
- 1 cup tomatoes, canned
- ¼ cup of water

Directions:

1. Mix tomato paste with harissa, peanut oil, and sesame oil. Whisk the mixture and mix it with sliced chicken breast.
2. After this, transfer the chicken in the Crock Pot in one layer.
3. Add water and close the lid.
4. Cook the chicken on High for 4 hours.

Apple Chicken Bombs

 **Servings: 7**   **Cooking Time: 4 hours**

Ingredients:

- 2 green apples, peeled and grated
- 12 oz. ground chicken
- 1 tsp minced garlic
- 1 tsp turmeric
- 1 egg
- 1 tbsp flour
- 1 tsp onion powder
- 1 tsp chili flakes
- ½ tsp salt
- 1 tsp garlic powder
- 1 tsp butter
- ½ cup panko bread crumbs

Directions:

1. Mix garlic, flour, turmeric, chili flakes, onion powder, garlic powder, and salt in a bowl.
2. Whisk in egg, ground chicken, and apple, then mix well.
3. Make small meatballs out of this mixture and coat them with breadcrumbs.
4. Grease the insert of the Crock Pot with butter.
5. Add the coated meatballs to the greased cooker.
6. Put the cooker's lid on and set the cooking time to 3 hours on High settings.
7. Flip the chicken balls and cook for another 1 hour on High setting.
8. Serve.

Almond-Stuffed Chicken

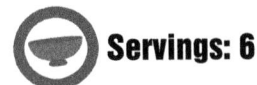 **Servings: 6**   **Cooking Time: 8 hours**

Ingredients:

- 1 ½ teaspoons butter
- 1/3 cup Boursin cheese or any herbed cheese of your choice
- ¼ cup slivered almonds, toasted and chopped
- 4 boneless chicken breasts, halved
- Salt and pepper to taste

Directions:

1. Line the bottom of the crockpot with foil.
2. Grease the foil with butter.
3. In a mixing bowl, mix together the cheese and almonds.
4. Cut a slit through the chicken breasts to create a pocket.
5. Season the chicken with salt and pepper to taste.
6. Spoon the cheese mixture into the slit on the chicken. Secure the slit with toothpicks.
7. Place the chicken in the foil-lined crockpot.
8. Cover with lid and cook on low for 8 hours or on high for 6 hours.

Asian Style Chicken

 **Servings: 4**   **Cooking Time: 8 hours**

Ingredients:

- 1 teaspoon hot sauce
- ¼ cup of soy sauce
- 1 teaspoon sesame oil
- 2 oz scallions, chopped
- ½ cup of orange juice
- 1 teaspoon ground coriander
- 1-pound chicken breast, skinless, boneless, roughly chopped

Directions:

1. Put all ingredients in the Crock Pot.
2. Close the lid and cook the meal on Low for 8 hours.
3. Then transfer the chicken and little amount of the chicken liquid in the bowls.

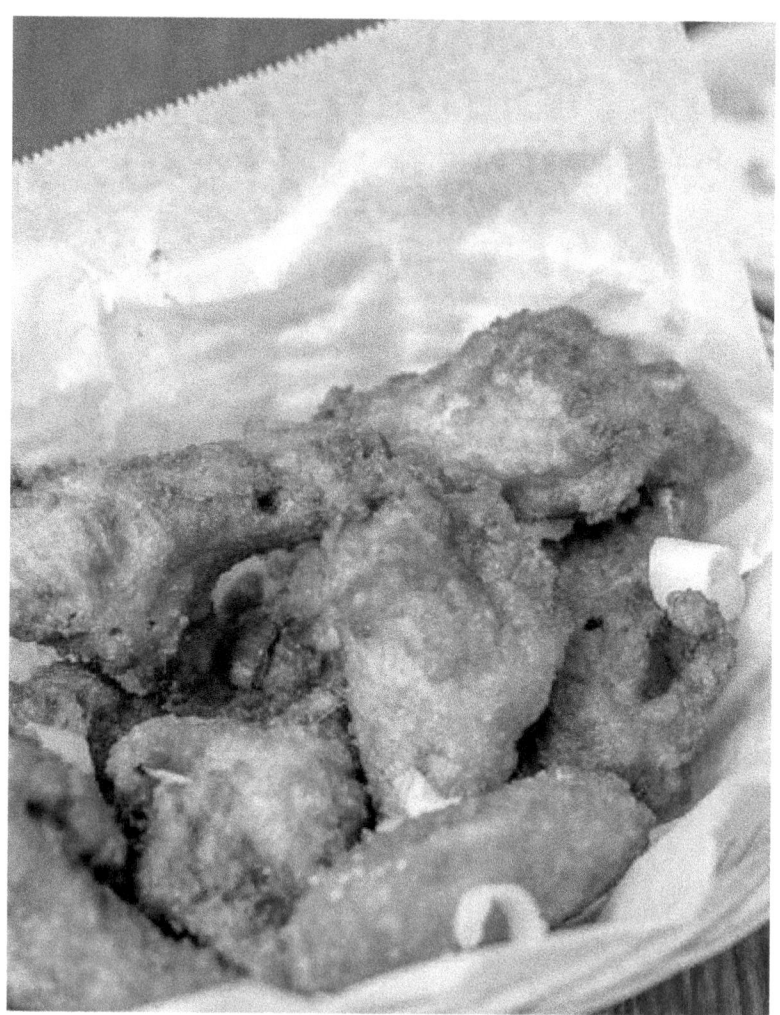

Banana Chicken

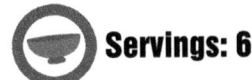 **Servings: 6**   **Cooking Time: 9 hours**

Ingredients:

- 2 bananas, chopped
- 2-pound whole chicken
- 1 tablespoon taco seasonings
- 1 tablespoon olive oil
- ½ cup of soy sauce
- ½ cup of water

Directions:

1. Fill the chicken with bananas and secure the whole.
2. Then rub the chicken with taco seasonings and brush with olive oil.
3. After this, pour water and soy sauce in the Crock Pot.
4. Add chicken and close the lid.
5. Cook it on Low for 9 hours.

Balsamic Turkey

 **Servings: 2**   **Cooking Time: 5 hours**

Ingredients:

- 1 pound turkey breast, skinless, boneless and cubed
- 1 tablespoon lemon juice
- 4 scallions, chopped
- 1 tablespoon balsamic vinegar
- 2 tablespoons avocado oil
- A pinch of salt and black pepper
- 1 tablespoon chives, chopped
- ½ cup chicken stock

Directions:

1. In your Crock Pot, mix the turkey with the lemon juice, scallions and the other ingredients, toss, put the lid on and cook on High for 5 hours.
2. Divide the mix between plates and serve right away.

Asparagus Chicken Salad

 **Servings: 4**   **Cooking Time: 4 hours**

Ingredients:

- 12 oz chicken fillet
- 7 oz asparagus, chopped, boiled
- 2 tablespoons mayonnaise
- 1 tablespoon lemon juice
- 1 teaspoon cayenne pepper
- 1 cup of water

Directions:

1. Put the chicken in the Crock Pot. Add water and close the lid.
2. Cook the chicken on high for 4 hours.
3. Then shred it and mix with chopped asparagus.
4. Add lemon juice, cayenne pepper, and mayonnaise.
5. Mix the salad.

Bacon Chicken Wings

 **Servings: 4**   **Cooking Time: 3 hours**

Ingredients:

- 4 chicken wings, boneless
- 4 bacon slices
- 1 tablespoon maple syrup
- ½ teaspoon ground black pepper
- ½ cup of water

Directions:

1. Sprinkle the chicken wings with ground black pepper and maple syrup.
2. Then wrap every chicken wing in the bacon and place it in the Crock Pot.
3. Add water and close the lid.
4. Cook the chicken wings in High for 3 hours.

Basic Shredded Chicken

 Servings: 12   **Cooking Time: 8 hours**

Ingredients:

- 6 pounds chicken breasts, bones and skin removed
- 1 teaspoon salt
- ½ teaspoon black pepper
- 5 cups homemade chicken broth
- 4 tablespoons butter

Directions:

1. Place all ingredients in the CrockPot.
2. Close the lid and cook on high for 6 hours or on low for 8 hours.
3. Shred the chicken meat using two forks.
4. Return to the CrockPot and cook on high for another 30 minutes.

Alfredo Chicken

 **Servings: 4** **Cooking Time: 2 hours 30 minutes**

Ingredients:

- 1 pound chicken breasts, skinless and boneless
- 4 tablespoons soft butter
- 1 cup chicken stock
- 2 cups heavy cream
- Salt and black pepper to the taste
- ½ teaspoon Italian seasoning
- ½ teaspoon garlic powder
- 1/3 cup parmesan, grated
- ½ pound rigatoni

Directions:

1. In your Crock Pot, mix chicken with butter, stock, cream, salt, pepper, garlic powder and Italian seasoning, stir, cover and cook on High for 2 hours.
2. Shred meat, return to Crock Pot, also add rigatoni and parmesan, cover and cook on High for 30 minutes more.
3. Divide between plates and serve.

African Chicken Meal

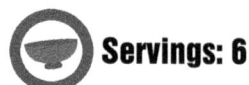 **Servings: 6**   **Cooking Time: 8 hours**

Ingredients:

- 13 oz. chicken breast
- 1 tsp peanut oil
- 1 tsp ground black pepper
- 1 tsp oregano
- 1 chili pepper
- 1 carrot
- 1 tbsp tomato sauce
- 1 cup tomatoes, canned
- 1 tbsp kosher salt
- ¼ tsp ground cardamom
- ½ tsp ground anise

Directions:

1. Rub the chicken breast with peanut oil then and sear for 1 minute per side in the skillet.
2. Transfer the chicken to the Crock Pot.
3. Add tomato sauce, salt, and all other ingredients to the cooker.
4. Put the cooker's lid on and set the cooking time to 8 hours on Low settings.
5. Serve.

Basil Chicken Saute

 **Servings: 4**   **Cooking Time: 7 hours**

Ingredients:

- 1 cup bell pepper
- 2 tomatoes, chopped
- 1 jalapeno pepper, chopped
- ½ cup of water
- 10 oz chicken fillet, chopped
- 1 teaspoon dried basil

Directions:

1. Pour water in the Crock Pot.
2. Add all remaining ingredients and close the lid.
3. Cook the chicken saute on Low for 7 hours.

Adobo Chicken Thighs

 Servings: 6

 Cooking Time: 8 hours

Ingredients:

- 5 garlic cloves, peeled and minced
- 6 white onions, peeled and diced
- 1 tbsp fresh ginger
- 1 oz. bay leaf
- 6 medium chicken thighs
- 5 tbsp soy sauce
- 1 tbsp apple cider vinegar
- 1 tsp white pepper
- ½ tsp sugar

Directions:

1. Arrange the medium-sized chicken thighs in the Crock Pot.
2. Mix onion with all other ingredients in a bowl.
3. Pour this onion mixture over the chicken thighs.
4. Put the cooker's lid on and set the cooking time to 8 hours on Low settings.
5. Serve warm.

Basil Chicken Wings

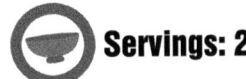 **Servings: 2**   **Cooking Time: 5 hours**

Ingredients:

- 1 pound chicken wings, halved
- 1 tablespoon olive oil
- 1 tablespoon honey
- 1 cup chicken stock
- A pinch of salt and black pepper
- 1 tablespoon basil, chopped
- ½ teaspoon cumin, ground

Directions:

1. In your Crock Pot, mix the chicken wings with the oil, honey and the other ingredients, toss, put the lid on and cook on High for 5 hours.
2. Divide the mix between plates and serve with a side salad.

41

Basil Chicken

 **Servings: 4**   **Cooking Time: 7 hours**

Ingredients:

- 2 tablespoons balsamic vinegar
- 1 cup of water
- 1 teaspoon dried basil
- 1 teaspoon dried oregano
- 1-pound chicken fillet, sliced
- 1 teaspoon mustard

Directions:

1. Mix chicken fillet with mustard and balsamic vinegar.
2. Add dried basil, oregano, and transfer in the Crock Pot.
3. Add water and close the lid.
4. Cook the chicken on low for 7 hours.

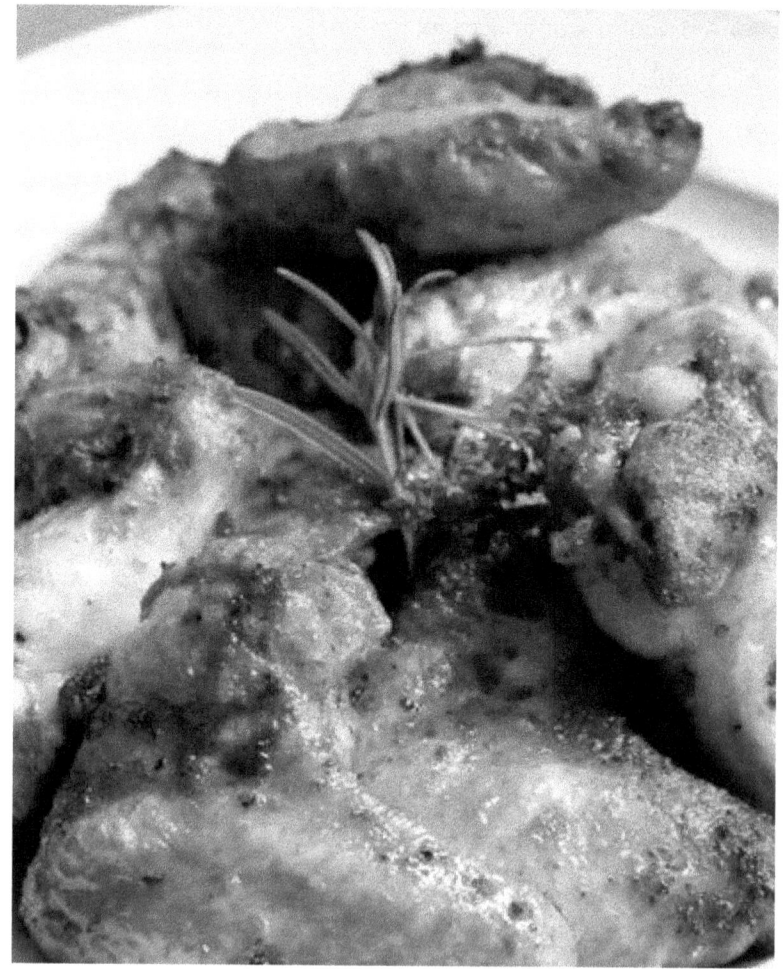

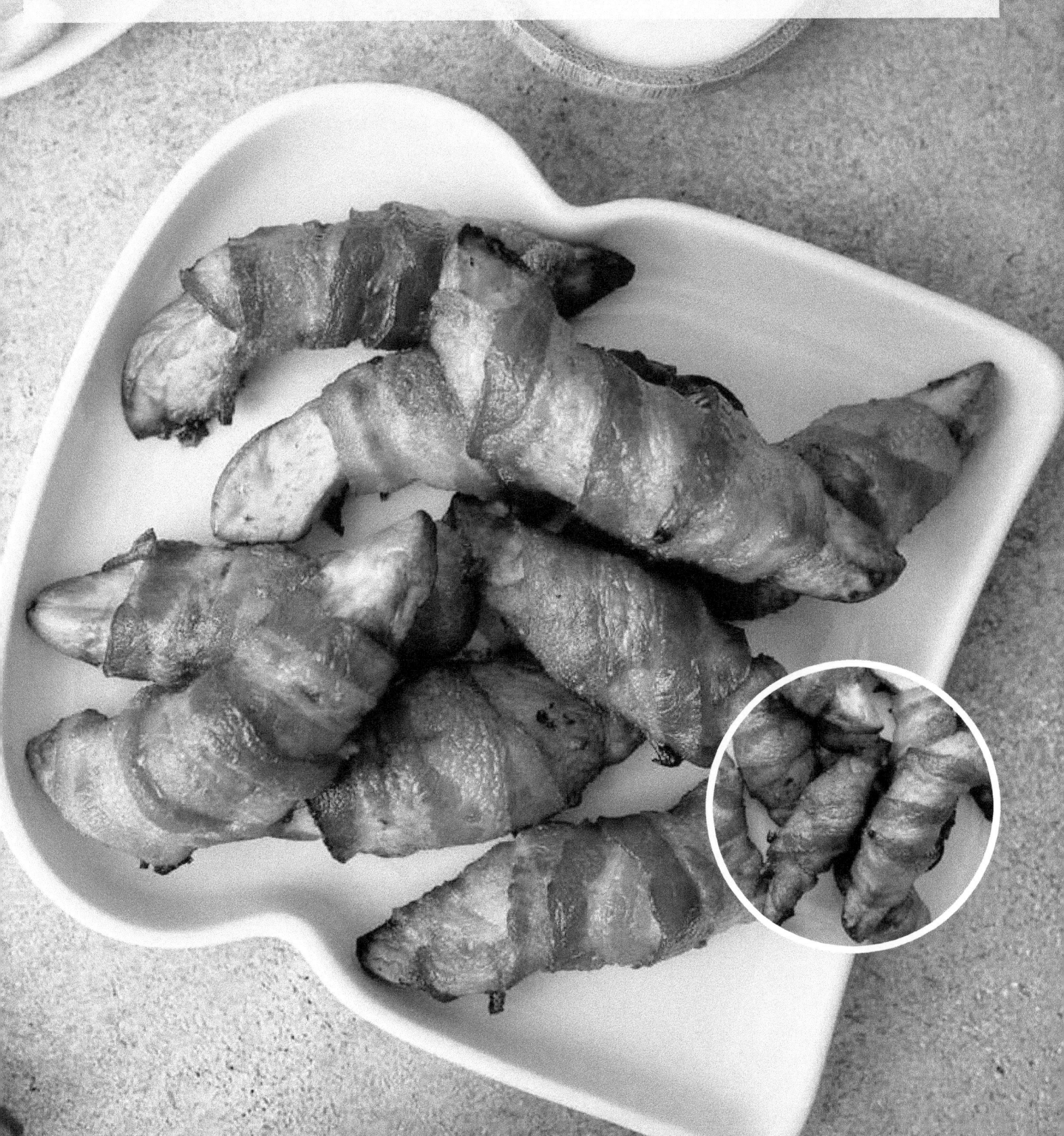

SIDE DISH RECIPES

Baked Potato

 **Servings: 6**

 Cooking Time: 8 hours

Ingredients:

- 6 large potatoes, peeled and cubed
- 3 oz. mushrooms, chopped
- 1 onion, chopped
- 1 tsp butter
- ½ tsp salt
- ½ tsp minced garlic
- 1 tsp sour cream
- ½ tsp turmeric
- 1 tsp olive oil

Directions:

1. Grease the insert of the Crock Pot with olive oil.
2. Toss in potatoes, onion, mushrooms, and rest of the ingredients.
3. Put the cooker's lid on and set the cooking time to 8 hours on Low settings.
4. Serve warm.

Balsamic Cauliflower

 **Servings: 2**   **Cooking Time: 5 hours**

Ingredients:

- 2 cups cauliflower florets
- ½ cup veggie stock
- 1 tablespoon balsamic vinegar
- 1 tablespoon lemon zest, grated
- 2 spring onions, chopped
- ¼ teaspoon sweet paprika
- Salt and black pepper to the taste
- 1 tablespoon dill, chopped

Directions:

1. In your Crock Pot, mix the cauliflower with the stock, vinegar and the other ingredients, toss, put the lid on and cook on Low for 5 hours.
2. Divide the cauliflower mix between plates and serve.

Baby Carrots and Parsnips Mix

 **Servings: 2**　　 **Cooking Time: 6 hours**

Ingredients:

- 1 tablespoon avocado oil
- 1 pound baby carrots, peeled
- ½ pound parsnips, peeled and cut into sticks
- 1 teaspoon sweet paprika
- ½ cup tomato paste
- ½ cup veggie stock
- ½ teaspoon chili powder
- A pinch of salt and black pepper
- 2 garlic cloves, minced
- 1 tablespoon dill, chopped

Directions:

1. Grease the Crock Pot with the oil and mix the carrots with the parsnips, paprika and the other ingredients inside.
2. Toss, put the lid on and cook on Low for 6 hours.
3. Divide everything between plates and serve as a side dish.

Asparagus and Mushroom Mix

 **Servings: 4**   **Cooking Time: 5 hours**

Ingredients:

- 2 pounds asparagus spears, cut into medium pieces
- 1 cup mushrooms, sliced
- A drizzle of olive oil
- Salt and black pepper to the taste
- 2 cups coconut milk
- 1 teaspoon Worcestershire sauce
- 5 eggs, whisked

Directions:

1. Grease your Crock Pot with the oil and spread asparagus and mushrooms on the bottom.
2. In a bowl, mix the eggs with milk, salt, pepper and Worcestershire sauce, whisk, pour into the Crock Pot, toss everything, cover and cook on Low for 6 hours.
3. Divide between plates and serve as a side dish.

Barley Mix

 **Servings: 2**   **Cooking Time: 6 hours**

Ingredients:

- 1 red onion, sliced
- ½ teaspoon sweet paprika
- ½ teaspoon turmeric powder
- 1 cup barley
- 1 cup veggie stock
- A pinch of salt and black pepper
- 1 garlic clove, minced

Directions:

1. In your Crock Pot, mix the barley with the onion, paprika and the other ingredients, toss, put the lid on and cook on Low for 6 hours.
2. Divide between plates and serve as a side dish.

Asparagus Mix

 **Servings: 2**   **Cooking Time: 2 hours**

Ingredients:

- 1 pound asparagus, trimmed and halved
- 1 red onion, sliced
- 2 garlic cloves, minced
- 1 cup veggie stock
- 1 tablespoon lemon juice
- A pinch of salt and black pepper
- ¼ cup parsley, chopped

Directions:

1. In your Crock Pot, mix the asparagus with the onion, garlic and the other ingredients, toss, put the lid on and cook on High for 2 hours.
2. Divide between plates and serve as a side dish.

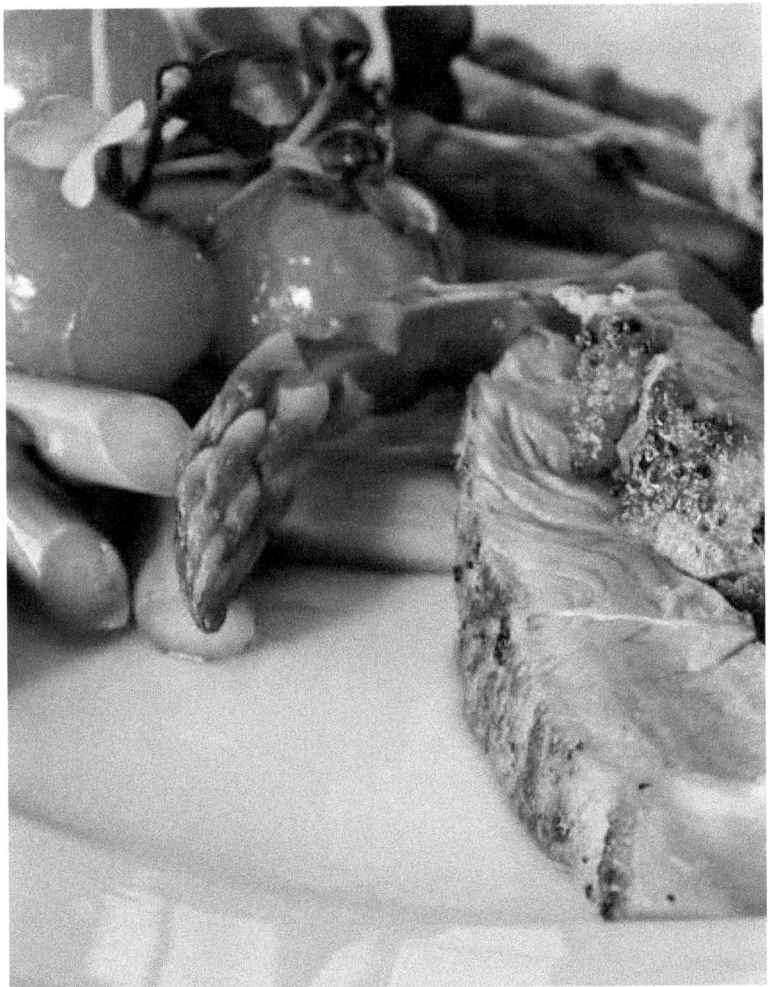

Beans Risotto

 **Servings: 6** **Cooking Time: 5 hours**

Ingredients:

- 1 lb. red kidney beans, soaked overnight and drained
- Salt to the taste
- 1 tsp olive oil
- 1 lb. smoked sausage, roughly chopped
- 1 yellow onion, chopped
- 1 celery stalk, chopped
- 4 garlic cloves, chopped
- 1 green bell pepper, chopped
- 1 tsp thyme, dried
- 2 bay leaves
- 5 cups of water
- 2 green onions, minced
- 2 tbsp parsley, minced

Directions:

1. Add red beans, oil, sausage, and rest of the ingredients to the Crock Pot.
2. Put the cooker's lid on and set the cooking time to 5 hours on Low settings.
3. Serve warm.

Beans, Carrots and Spinach Salad

 **Servings: 6** **Cooking Time: 7 hours**

Ingredients:

- 1 and ½ cups northern beans
- 1 yellow onion, chopped
- 5 carrots, chopped
- 2 garlic cloves, minced
- ½ teaspoon oregano, dried
- Salt and black pepper to the taste
- 4 and ½ cups chicken stock
- 5 ounces baby spinach
- 2 teaspoons lemon peel, grated
- 1 avocado, peeled, pitted and chopped
- 3 tablespoons lemon juice
- ¾ cup feta cheese, crumbled
- 1/3 cup pistachios, chopped

Directions:

1. In your Crock Pot, mix beans with onion, carrots, garlic, oregano, salt, pepper and stock, stir, cover and cook on Low for 7 hours.
2. Drain beans and veggies, transfer them to a salad bowl, add baby spinach, lemon peel, avocado, lemon juice, pistachios and cheese, toss, divide between plates and serve as a side dish.

Beans and Red Peppers

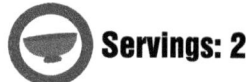 **Servings: 2**   **Cooking Time: 2 hours**

Ingredients:

- 2 cups green beans, halved
- 1 red bell pepper, cut into strips
- Salt and black pepper to the taste
- 1 tbsp olive oil
- 1 and ½ tbsp honey mustard

Directions:

1. Add green beans, honey mustard, red bell pepper, oil, salt, and black to Crock Pot.
2. Put the cooker's lid on and set the cooking time to 2 hours on High settings.
3. Serve warm.

Bean Medley

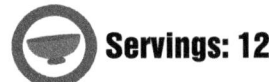 **Servings: 12**   **Cooking Time: 5 hours**

Ingredients:

- 2 celery ribs, chopped
- 1 and ½ cups ketchup
- 1 green bell pepper, chopped
- 1 yellow onion, chopped
- 1 sweet red pepper, chopped
- ½ cup brown sugar
- ½ cup Italian dressing
- ½ cup water
- 1 tablespoon cider vinegar
- 2 bay leaves
- 16 ounces kidney beans, drained
- Salt and black pepper to the taste
- 15 ounces canned black-eyed peas, drained
- 15 ounces canned northern beans, drained
- 15 ounces canned corn, drained
- 15 ounces canned lima beans, drained
- 15 ounces canned black beans, drained

Directions:

1. In your Crock Pot, mix celery with ketchup, red and green bell pepper, onion, sugar, Italian dressing, water, vinegar, bay leaves, kidney beans, black-eyed peas, northern beans, corn, lima beans and black beans, stir, cover and cook on Low for 5 hours.
2. Divide between plates and serve as a side dish.

Beets and Carrots

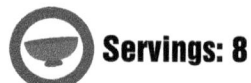 **Servings: 8**   **Cooking Time: 7 hours**

Ingredients:

- 2 tablespoons stevia
- ¾ cup pomegranate juice
- 2 teaspoons ginger, grated
- 2 and ½ pounds beets, peeled and cut into wedges
- 12 ounces carrots, cut into medium wedges

Directions:

1. In your Crock Pot, mix beets with carrots, ginger, stevia and pomegranate juice, toss, cover and cook on Low for 7 hours.
2. Divide between plates and serve as a side dish.

Balsamic-Glazed Beets

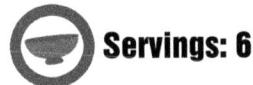 **Servings: 6**   **Cooking Time: 2 hours**

Ingredients:

- 1 lb. beets, sliced
- 5 oz. orange juice
- 3 oz. balsamic vinegar
- 3 tbsp almonds
- 6 oz. goat cheese
- 1 tsp minced garlic
- 1 tsp olive oil

Directions:

1. Toss the beets with balsamic vinegar, orange juice, and olive oil in the insert of Crock Pot.
2. Put the cooker's lid on and set the cooking time to 7 hours on Low settings.
3. Toss goat cheese with minced garlic and almonds in a bowl.
4. Spread this cheese garlic mixture over the beets.
5. Put the cooker's lid on and set the cooking time to 10 minutes on High settings.
6. Serve warm.

Bbq Beans

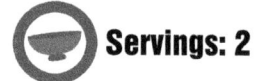 **Servings: 2**   **Cooking Time: 8 hours**

Ingredients:

- ¼ pound navy beans, soaked overnight and drained
- 1 cup bbq sauce
- 1 tablespoon sugar
- 1 tablespoon ketchup
- 1 tablespoon water
- 1 tablespoon apple cider vinegar
- 1 tablespoon olive oil
- 1 tablespoon soy sauce

Directions:

1. In your Crock Pot, mix the beans with the sauce, sugar and the other ingredients, toss, put the lid on and cook on Low for 8 hours.
2. Divide between plates and serve as a side dish.

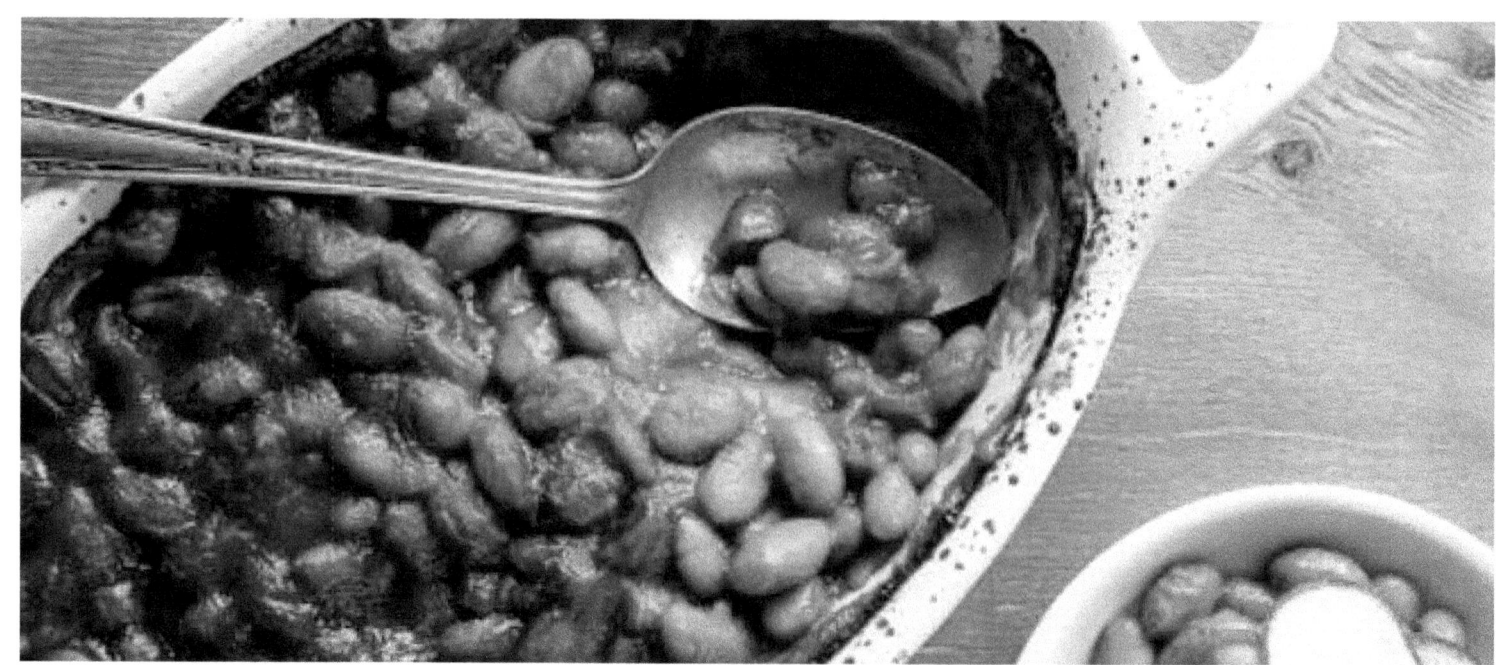

Bacon Potatoes Mix

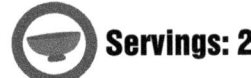 **Servings: 2**   **Cooking Time: 6 hours**

Ingredients:

- 2 sweet potatoes, peeled and cut into wedges
- 1 tablespoon balsamic vinegar
- ½ tablespoon sugar
- A pinch of salt and black pepper
- ¼ teaspoon sage, dried
- A pinch of thyme, dried
- 1 tablespoon olive oil
- ½ cup veggie stock
- 2 bacon slices, cooked and crumbled

Directions:

1. In your Crock Pot, mix the potatoes with the vinegar, sugar and the other ingredients, toss, put the lid on and cook on Low for 6 hours
2. Divide between plates and serve as a side dish.

Balsamic Okra Mix

 Servings: 4   Cooking Time: 2 hours

Ingredients:

- 2 cups okra, sliced
- 1 cup cherry tomatoes, halved
- 1 tablespoon olive oil
- ½ teaspoon turmeric powder
- ½ cup canned tomatoes, crushed
- 2 tablespoons balsamic vinegar
- 2 tablespoons basil, chopped
- 1 tablespoon thyme, chopped

Directions:

1. In your Crock Pot, mix the okra with the tomatoes, crushed tomatoes and the other ingredients, toss, put the lid on and cook on High for 2 hours.
2. Divide between plates and serve as a side dish.

Apples and Potatoes

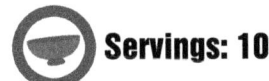 **Servings: 10**   **Cooking Time: 7 hours**

Ingredients:

- 2 green apples, cored and cut into wedges
- 3 pounds sweet potatoes, peeled and cut into medium wedges
- 1 cup coconut cream
- ½ cup dried cherries
- 1 cup apple butter
- 1 and ½ teaspoon pumpkin pie spice

Directions:

1. In your Crock Pot, mix sweet potatoes with green apples, cream, cherries, apple butter and spice, toss, cover and cook on Low for 7 hours.
2. Toss, divide between plates and serve as a side dish.

Asian Sesame Asparagus

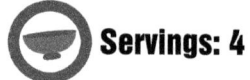 **Servings: 4**   **Cooking Time: 4 hours**

Ingredients:

- 1 tbsp sesame seeds
- 1 tsp miso paste
- ¼ cup of soy sauce
- 1 cup fish stock
- 8 oz. asparagus
- 1 tsp salt
- 1 tsp chili flakes
- 1 tsp oregano
- 1 cup of water

Directions:

1. Fill the insert of the Crock Pot with water and add asparagus.
2. Put the cooker's lid on and set the cooking time to 3 hours on High settings.
3. During this time, mix miso paste with soy sauce, fish stock, and sesame seeds in a suitable bowl.
4. Stir in oregano, chili flakes, and salt, then mix well.
5. Drain the slow-cooked asparagus then return it to the Crock Pot.
6. Pour the miso-stock mixture over the asparagus.
7. Put the cooker's lid on and set the cooking time to 1 hour on High settings.
8. Serve warm.

Beets Salad

 **Servings: 12**   **Cooking Time: 7 hours**

Ingredients:

- 5 beets, peeled and sliced
- ¼ cup balsamic vinegar
- 1/3 cup honey
- 1 tbsp rosemary, chopped
- 2 tbsp olive oil
- Salt and black pepper to the taste
- 2 garlic cloves, minced

Directions:

1. Add beets, oil, vinegar, salt, black pepper, honey, garlic, and rosemary to the Crock Pot.
2. Put the cooker's lid on and set the cooking time to 7 hours on Low settings.
3. Serve warm.

Beets Side Salad

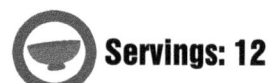

Ingredients:

- 5 beets, peeled and sliced
- ¼ cup balsamic vinegar
- 1/3 cup honey
- 1 tablespoon rosemary, chopped
- 2 tablespoons olive oil
- Salt and black pepper to the taste
- 2 garlic cloves, minced

Directions:

1. In your Crock Pot, mix beets with vinegar, honey, oil, salt, pepper, rosemary and garlic, cover and cook on Low for 7 hours.
2. Divide between plates and serve as a side dish.

Berry Wild Rice

 **Servings: 4**   **Cooking Time: 5 hours 30 minutes**

Ingredients:

- 2 cups wild rice
- 4 cups of water
- 1 tsp salt
- 6 oz. cherries, dried
- 1 tbsp chives
- 1 tbsp butter
- 2 tbsp heavy cream

Directions:

1. Add wild rice, salt, water, and dried cherries to the Crock Pot.
2. Put the cooker's lid on and set the cooking time to 5 hours on High settings.
3. Stir in cream and butter, then cover again to cook for 30 minutes on the low setting.
4. Serve.

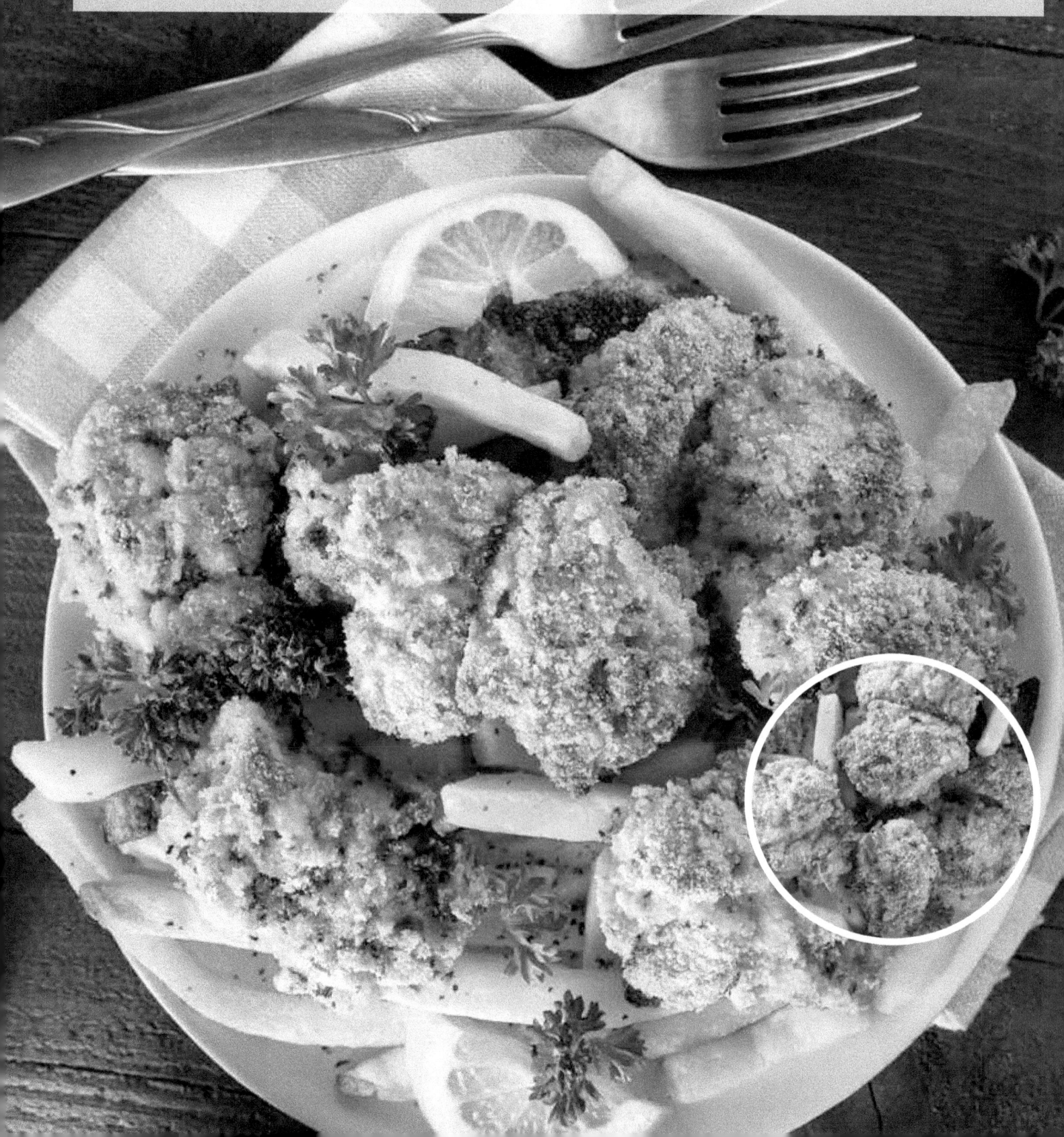

SNACK RECIPES

Almond, Zucchini, Parmesan Snack

 **Servings: 6**   **Cooking Time: 1 hour 40 minutes**

Ingredients:

- 3 eggs, organic
- 2 zucchinis, thinly sliced
- 1 cup almonds, ground
- 1 cup Parmesan cheese, grated
- Salt and pepper to taste
- Olive oil
- 1 teaspoon oregano
- 1 cup almond flour

Directions:

1. Wash, clean, and slice the zucchini. Salt and set aside on a paper towel.
2. On a plate, combine Parmesan cheese, almonds, oregano, salt, and pepper and set aside.
3. On another shallow plate, spread the almond flour. In a bowl, beat eggs with salt and pepper. Start by dipping zucchini rounds in flour, dip in the eggs, then dredge in almond mixture, pressing on them to coat.
4. Pour olive oil in Crock-Pot and add the zucchini slices; cover and cook for 1 ½ hours on HIGH.
5. Serve hot.

Basic Pepper Salsa

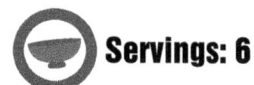 **Servings: 6**   **Cooking Time: 5 hours**

Ingredients:

- 7 cups tomatoes, chopped
- 1 green bell pepper, chopped
- 1 red bell pepper, chopped
- 2 yellow onions, chopped
- 4 jalapenos, chopped
- ¼ cup apple cider vinegar
- 1 tsp coriander, ground
- 1 tbsp cilantro, chopped
- 3 tbsp basil, chopped
- Salt and black pepper to the taste

Directions:

1. Add jalapenos, tomatoes and all other ingredients to the Crock Pot.
2. Put the cooker's lid on and set the cooking time to 5 hours on Low settings.
3. Mix gently and serve.

Artichoke & Spinach Mash

 **Servings: 8**   **Cooking Time: 2 hours 25 minutes**

Ingredients:

- 1 ½ cups frozen spinach, thawed
- 2 cans artichoke hearts, drained and chopped
- 1 cup sour cream
- ¾ cup Parmesan cheese, freshly grated
- ½ cup Feta cheese, crumbled
- 1 cup cream cheese
- 2 green onions, diced
- 2 cloves garlic, minced
- ¼ teaspoon ground pepper

Directions:

1. Add artichoke hearts, spinach, and other ingredients to Crock-Pot.
2. Stir until all ingredients are well combined. Top with cream cheese.
3. Cover and cook on LOW for 2 hours and 15 minutes. Before serving, give dish a good stir.

Apple Chutney

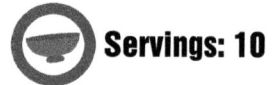 **Servings: 10** **Cooking Time: 9 hours**

Ingredients:

- 1 cup wine vinegar
- 4 oz. brown sugar
- 2 lbs. apples, chopped
- 4 oz. onion, chopped
- 1 jalapeno pepper
- 1 tsp ground cardamom
- ½ tsp ground cinnamon
- 1 tsp chili flakes

Directions:

1. Mix brown sugar with wine vinegar in the Crock Pot.
2. Put the cooker's lid on and set the cooking time to 1 hour on High settings.
3. Add chopped apples and all other ingredients to the cooker.
4. Put the cooker's lid on and set the cooking time to 8 hours on Low settings.
5. Mix well and mash the mixture with a fork.
6. Serve.

Apple Jelly Sausage Snack

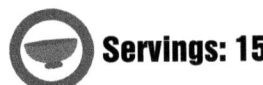 Servings: 15   Cooking Time: 2 hours

Ingredients:

- 2 pounds sausages, sliced
- 18 ounces apple jelly
- 9 ounces Dijon mustard

Directions:

1. Place sausage slices in your Crock Pot, add apple jelly and mustard, toss to coat well, cover and cook on Low for 2 hours.
2. Divide into bowls and serve as a snack.

Artichoke Dip

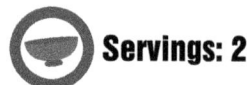 **Servings: 2**   **Cooking Time: 2 hours**

Ingredients:

- 2 ounces canned artichoke hearts, drained and chopped
- 2 ounces heavy cream
- 2 tablespoons mayonnaise
- ¼ cup mozzarella, shredded
- 2 green onions, chopped
- ½ teaspoon garam masala
- Cooking spray

Directions:

1. Grease your Crock Pot with the cooking spray, and mix the artichokes with the cream, mayo and the other ingredients inside.
2. Stir, cover, cook on Low for 2 hours, divide into bowls and serve as a party dip.

Bacon Fingerling Potatoes

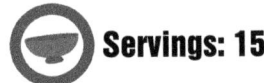 Servings: 15   Cooking Time: 8 hours

Ingredients:

- 2 lb. fingerling potatoes
- 8 oz. bacon
- 1 tsp onion powder
- 1 tsp chili powder
- 1 tsp garlic powder
- 1 tsp paprika
- 3 tbsp butter
- 1 tsp dried dill
- 1 tbsp rosemary

Directions:

1. Grease the base of your Crock Pot with butter.
2. Spread the fingerling potatoes in the buttered cooker.
3. Mix all the spices, herbs, and bacon in a bowl.
4. Spread bacon-spice mixture over the lingering potatoes.
5. Put the cooker's lid on and set the cooking time to 8 hours on Low settings.
6. Serve warm.

BBQ Chicken Dip

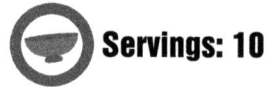 **Servings: 10**   **Cooking Time: 1 hour 30 minutes**

Ingredients:

- 1 and ½ cups bbq sauce
- 1 small red onion, chopped
- 24 ounces cream cheese, cubed
- 2 cups rotisserie chicken, shredded
- 3 bacon slices, cooked and crumbled
- 1 plum tomato, chopped
- ½ cup cheddar cheese, shredded
- 1 tablespoon green onions, chopped

Directions:

1. In your Crock Pot, mix bbq sauce with onion, cream cheese, rotisserie chicken, bacon, tomato, cheddar and green onions, stir, cover and cook on Low for 1 hour and 30 minutes.
2. Divide into bowls and serve.

Apple Wedges with Peanuts

 **Servings: 5**   **Cooking Time: 2 hours**

Ingredients:

- 1 tbsp peanut butter
- 3 tbsp peanut, crushed
- 6 green apples, cut into wedges
- ½ tsp cinnamon
- 1 tbsp butter
- 2 tsp water
- 1 tsp lemon zest
- 1 tsp lemon juice

Directions:

1. Toss the peanuts with peanut butter, butter, lemon zest, cinnamon, and lemon juice in a bowl.
2. Stir in apple wedges and mix well to coat them.
3. Transfer the apple to the Crock Pot along with 2 tsp water.
4. Put the cooker's lid on and set the cooking time to 2 hours on High settings.
5. Serve.

Apple Sausage Snack

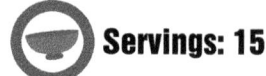 Servings: 15   Cooking Time: 2 hours

Ingredients:

- 2 lbs. sausages, sliced
- 18 oz. apple jelly
- 9 oz. Dijon mustard

Directions:

1. Add sausage slices, apple jelly, and mustard to the Crock Pot.
2. Put the cooker's lid on and set the cooking time to 2 hours on Low settings.
3. Serve fresh.

Bean Dip

 Servings: 56   Cooking Time: 3 hours

Ingredients:

- 16 ounces Mexican cheese
- 5 ounces canned green chilies
- 16 ounces canned refried beans
- 2 pounds tortilla chips
- Cooking spray

Directions:

1. Grease your Crock Pot with cooking spray, line it, add Mexican cheese, green chilies and refried beans, stir, cover and cook on Low for 3 hours.
2. Divide into bowls and serve with tortilla chips on the side.

Apple Dip

 **Servings: 8**   **Cooking Time: 1 hour 30 minutes**

Ingredients:

- 5 apples, peeled and chopped
- ½ teaspoon cinnamon powder
- 12 ounces jarred caramel sauce
- A pinch of nutmeg, ground

Directions:

1. In your Crock Pot, mix apples with cinnamon, caramel sauce and nutmeg, stir, cover and cook on High for 1 hour and 30 minutes.
2. Divide into bowls and serve.

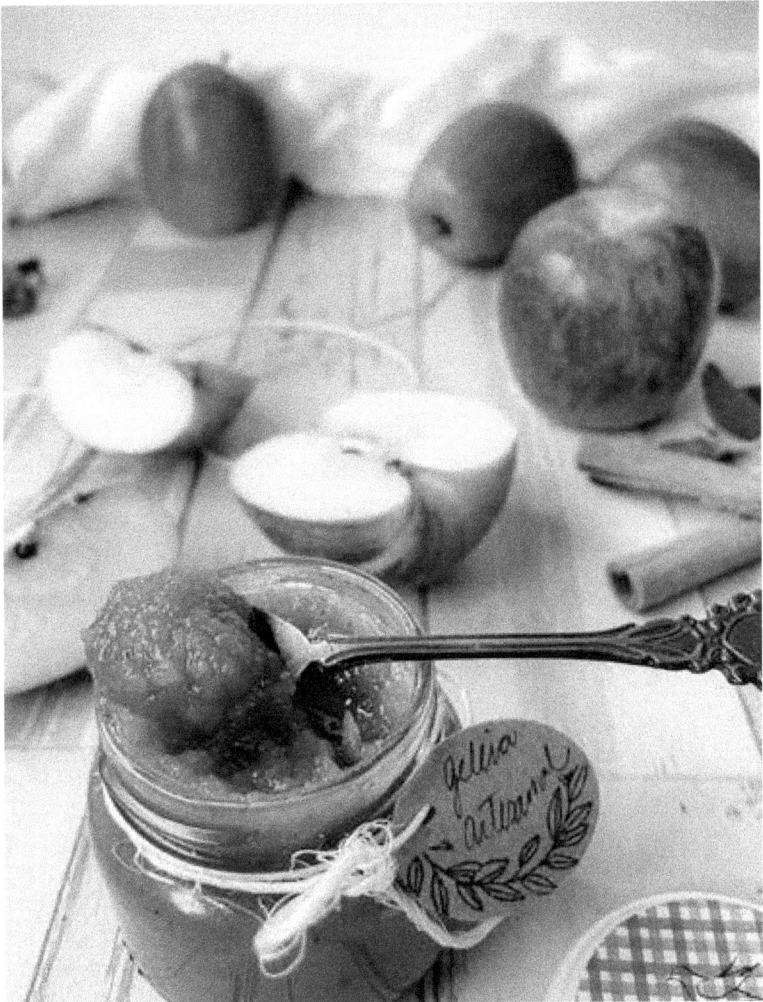

Apple and Carrot Dip

 **Servings: 2**   **Cooking Time: 6 hours**

Ingredients:

- 2 cups apples, peeled, cored and chopped
- 1 cup carrots, peeled and grated
- ¼ teaspoon cloves, ground
- ¼ teaspoon ginger powder
- 1 tablespoon lemon juice
- ½ tablespoon lemon zest, grated
- ½ cup coconut cream
- ¼ teaspoon nutmeg, ground

Directions:

1. In your Crock Pot, mix the apples with the carrots, cloves and the other ingredients, toss, put the lid on and cook on Low for 6 hours.
2. Bend using an immersion blender, divide into bowls and serve.

Almond Spread

 **Servings: 2**   **Cooking Time: 8 hours**

Ingredients:

- ¼ cup almonds
- 1 cup heavy cream
- ½ teaspoon nutritional yeast flakes
- A pinch of salt and black pepper

Directions:

1. In your Crock Pot, mix the almonds with the cream and the other ingredients, toss, put the lid on and cook on Low for 8 hours.
2. Transfer to a blender, pulse well, divide into bowls and serve.

"Pumpkin Pie" with Almond Meal

 **Servings: 8**   **Cooking Time: 3 hours 15 minutes**

Ingredients:

- 4 tablespoons coconut oil
- 1 ¾ cups almond meal
- 2 cups pure pumpkin
- 1 teaspoon pumpkin pie spice
- Natural sweetener of your choice, to taste
- 3 eggs
- ½ teaspoon of cloves, ground
- 1 ¼ teaspoon baking powder
- 1 ¼ teaspoon baking soda
- 1 teaspoon cinnamon, ground
- Sea salt to taste

Directions:

1. In a mixing bowl, beat together coconut oil and sweetener of your choice. Add eggs and whisk until well combined.
2. Add the pumpkin and spices, almond flour, baking powder, baking soda and sea salt. Pour batter into a greased baking dish and place it in Crock-Pot. Cover with lid and cook on HIGH for 3 hours.
3. When ready, let it cool down and serve.

Almond Bowls

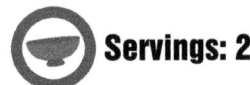 **Servings: 2**   **Cooking Time: 4 hours**

Ingredients:

- 1 tablespoon cinnamon powder
- 1 cup sugar
- 2 cups almonds
- ½ cup water
- ½ teaspoons vanilla extract

Directions:

1. In your Crock Pot, mix the almonds with the cinnamon and the other ingredients, toss, put the lid on and cook on Low for 4 hours.
2. Divide into bowls and serve as a snack.

Almond Buns

 **Servings: 6**   **Cooking Time: 20 minutes**

Ingredients:

- 3 cups almond flour
- 5 tablespoons butter
- 1 ½ teaspoons sweetener of your choice (optional)
- 2 eggs
- 1 ½ teaspoons baking powder

Directions:

1. In a mixing bowl, combine the dry ingredients.
2. In another bowl, whisk the eggs.
3. Add melted butter to mixture and mix well.
4. Divide almond mixture equally into 6 parts.
5. Grease the bottom of Crock-Pot and place in 6 almond buns.
6. Cover and cook on HIGH for 2 to 2 ½ hours or LOW for 4 to 4 ½ hours. Serve hot.

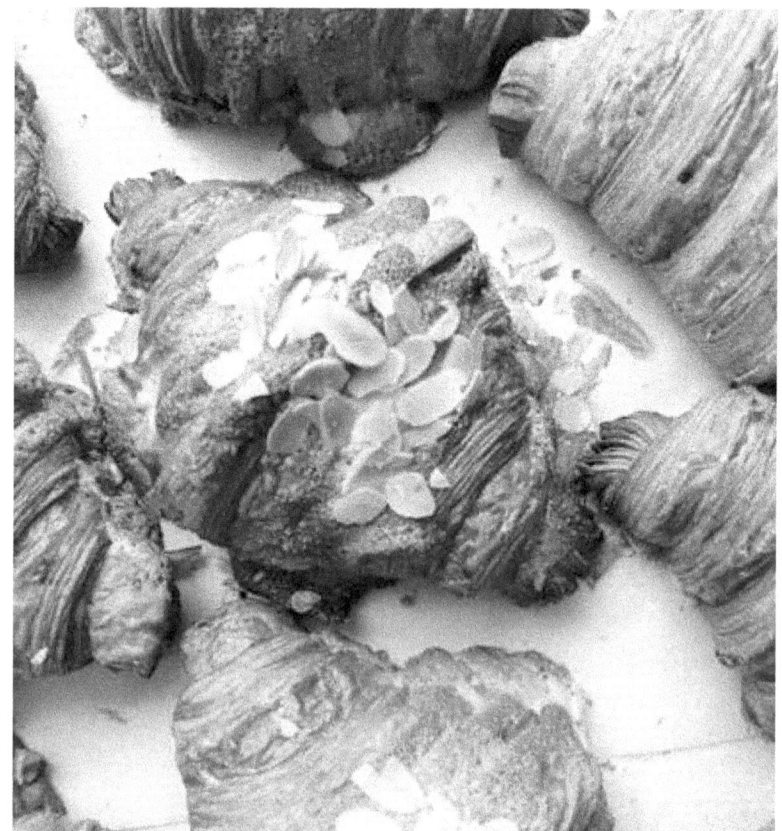

Bean Pesto Dip

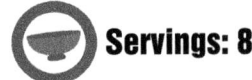 **Servings: 8**   **Cooking Time: 6 hours**

Ingredients:

- 10 oz. refried beans
- 1 tbsp pesto sauce
- 1 tsp salt
- 7 oz. Cheddar cheese, shredded
- 1 tsp paprika
- 1 cup of salsa
- 4 tbsp sour cream
- 2-oz. cream cheese
- 1 tsp dried dill

Directions:

1. Mix pesto with salt, salsa, sour cream, dill, beans, cheese, paprika, and cream cheese in the Crock Pot.
2. Put the cooker's lid on and set the cooking time to 6 hours on Low settings.
3. Once Crock Pot, blend the mixture using a hand blender.
4. Serve fresh.

Bean Salsa Salad

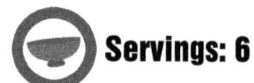 **Servings: 6**   **Cooking Time: 4 hours**

Ingredients:

- 1 tbsp soy sauce
- ½ tsp cumin, ground
- 1 cup canned black beans
- 1 cup of salsa
- 6 cups romaine lettuce leaves
- ½ cup avocado, peeled, pitted and mashed

Directions:

1. Add black beans, cumin, soy sauce, and salsa to the Crock Pot.
2. Put the cooker's lid on and set the cooking time to 4 hours on Low settings.
3. Transfer the beans to a salad bowl and toss in lettuce leaves, and mashed avocado.
4. Mix well then serve.

Beans Spread

 **Servings: 2**   **Cooking Time: 6 hours**

Ingredients:

- 1 cup canned black beans, drained
- 2 tablespoons tahini paste
- ½ teaspoon balsamic vinegar
- ¼ cup veggie stock
- ½ tablespoon olive oil

Directions:

1. In your Crock Pot, mix the beans with the tahini paste and the other ingredients, toss, put the lid on and cook on Low for 6 hours.
2. Transfer to your food processor, blend well, divide into bowls and serve.

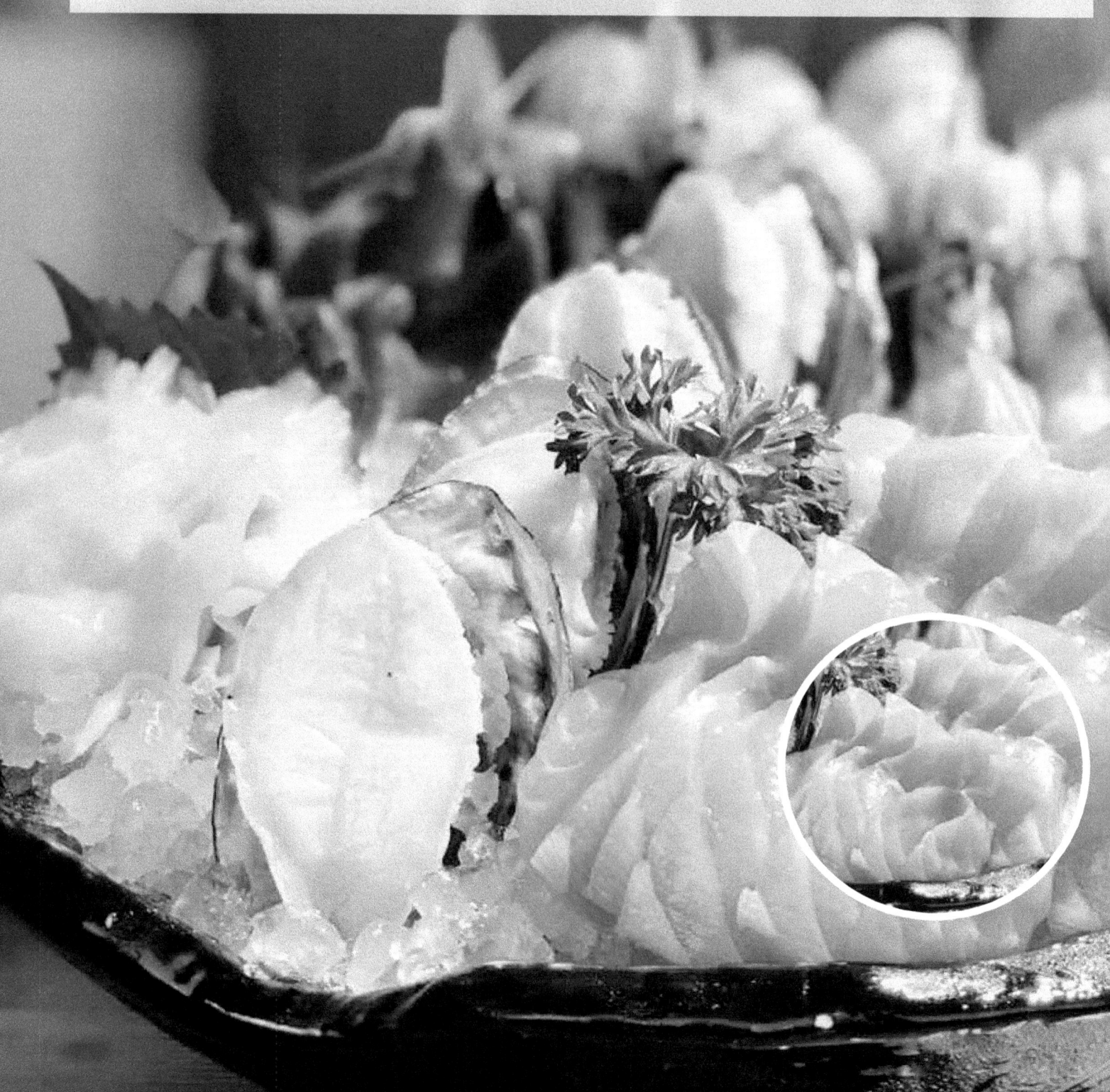

FISH & SEAFOOD RECIPES

Baked Cod

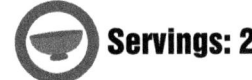 **Servings: 2**   **Cooking Time: 5 hours**

Ingredients:

- 2 cod fillets
- 2 teaspoons cream cheese
- 2 tablespoons bread crumbs
- 1 teaspoon salt
- ½ teaspoon cayenne pepper
- 2 oz Mozzarella, shredded

Directions:

1. Sprinkle the cod fillets with cayenne pepper and salt.
2. Put the fish in the Crock Pot.
3. Then top it with cream cheese, bread crumbs, and Mozzarella.
4. Close the lid and cook the meal for 5 hours on Low.

Almond-Crusted Tilapia

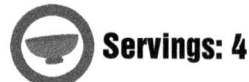 **Servings: 4**   **Cooking Time: 4 hours**

Ingredients:

- 2 tablespoons olive oil
- 1 cup chopped almonds
- ¼ cup ground flaxseed
- 4 tilapia fillets
- Salt and pepper to taste

Directions:

1. Line the bottom of the crockpot with a foil.
2. Grease the foil with the olive oil.
3. In a mixing bowl, combine the almonds and flaxseed.
4. Season the tilapia with salt and pepper to taste.
5. Dredge the tilapia fillets with the almond and flaxseed mixture.
6. Place neatly in the foil-lined crockpot.
7. Close the lid and cook on high for 2 hours and on low for 4 hours.

Balsamic-Glazed Salmon

 **Servings: 7**   **Cooking Time: 1.5 hours**

Ingredients:

- 5 tbsp brown sugar
- 2 tbsp sesame seeds
- 1 tbsp balsamic vinegar
- 1 tbsp butter
- 3 tbsp water
- 1 tsp salt
- ½ tsp ground black pepper
- 1 tsp ground paprika
- 1 tsp turmeric
- ¼ tsp fresh rosemary
- 1 tsp olive oil
- 21 oz salmon fillet

Directions:

1. Whisk rosemary, black pepper, salt, turmeric, and paprika in a small bowl.
2. Rub the salmon fillet with this spice's mixture.
3. Grease a suitable pan with olive oil and place it over medium-high heat.
4. Place the spiced salmon fillet in the hot pan and sear it for 3 minutes per side.
5. Add butter, sesame seeds, brown sugar, balsamic vinegar, and water to the insert of the Crock Pot.
6. Put the cooker's lid on and set the cooking time to 30 minutes on High settings.
7. Stir this sugar mixture occasionally.
8. Place the salmon fillet in the Crock Pot.
9. Put the cooker's lid on and set the cooking time to 1 hour on Low settings.
10. Serve warm.

Basil Octopus

 **Servings: 3**   **Cooking Time: 4 hours**

Ingredients:

- 12 oz octopus, chopped
- 1 orange, chopped
- 1 teaspoon dried basil
- ½ cup of water
- 1 teaspoon butter

Directions:

1. Put all ingredients in the Crock Pot.
2. Close the lid and cook the octopus on Low for 4 hours or until it is soft.

Balsamic Trout

 Servings: 2   **Cooking Time: 3 hours**

Ingredients:

- 1 pound trout fillets, boneless
- ½ cup chicken stock
- 2 garlic cloves, minced
- 2 tablespoons balsamic vinegar
- ½ teaspoon cumin, ground
- Salt and black pepper to the taste
- 1 tablespoon parsley, chopped
- 1 tablespoon olive oil

Directions:

1. In your Crock Pot, mix the trout with the stock, garlic and the other ingredients, toss gently, put the lid on and cook on High for 3 hours.
2. Divide the mix between plates and serve.

Bacon-Wrapped Shrimps

 Servings: 4 Cooking Time: 2 hours

Ingredients:

- 2 tablespoons butter, melted
- 30 large shrimps, shelled
- ½ teaspoon garlic powder
- Salt and pepper to taste
- 15 strips bacon, cut lengthwise

Directions:

1. Line the crockpot bottom with foil.
2. Pour the butter into the crockpot.
3. Marinate the shrimps with garlic powder, salt and pepper. Allow to stay in the fridge for 30 minutes.
4. Wrap the shrimps with bacon and arrange in the crockpot.
5. Close the lid and cook on low for 2 hours or on high for 45 minutes.
6. Be sure to flip the shrimps to sear the other side.

Bacon-Wrapped Salmon

 **Servings: 2**   **Cooking Time: 6 hours**

Ingredients:

- 2 salmon fillets
- 1 teaspoon liquid honey
- ¼ teaspoon dried thyme
- 2 bacon slices
- 1 teaspoon sunflower oil
- ¼ cup of water

Directions:

1. Sprinkle the salmon fillets with dried thyme and wrap in the bacon.
2. Then pour water in the Crock Pot.
3. Add sunflower oil and honey.
4. Then add wrapped salmon and close the lid.
5. Cook the meal on low for 6 hours.

Balsamic Tuna

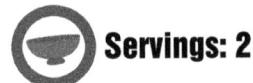 **Servings: 2**   **Cooking Time: 3 hours**

Ingredients:

- 1 pound tuna fillets, boneless and roughly cubed
- 1 tablespoon balsamic vinegar
- 3 garlic cloves, minced
- 1 tablespoon avocado oil
- ¼ cup chicken stock
- 1 tablespoon hives, chopped
- A pinch of salt and black pepper

Directions:

1. In your Crock Pot, mix the tuna with the garlic, vinegar and the other ingredients, toss, put the lid on and cook on Low for 3 hours.
2. Divide the mix into bowls and serve.

Basil Cod and Olives

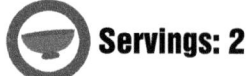 **Servings: 2**   **Cooking Time: 3 hours**

Ingredients:

- 1 pound cod fillets, boneless
- 1 cup black olives, pitted and halved
- ½ tablespoon tomato paste
- 1 tablespoon basil, chopped
- ¼ cup chicken stock
- 1 red onion, sliced
- 1 tablespoon lime juice
- 1 tablespoon chives, chopped
- Salt and black pepper to the taste

Directions:

1. In your Crock Pot, mix the cod with the olives, basil and the other ingredients, toss, put the lid on and cook on Low for 3 hours.
2. Divide everything between plates and serve.

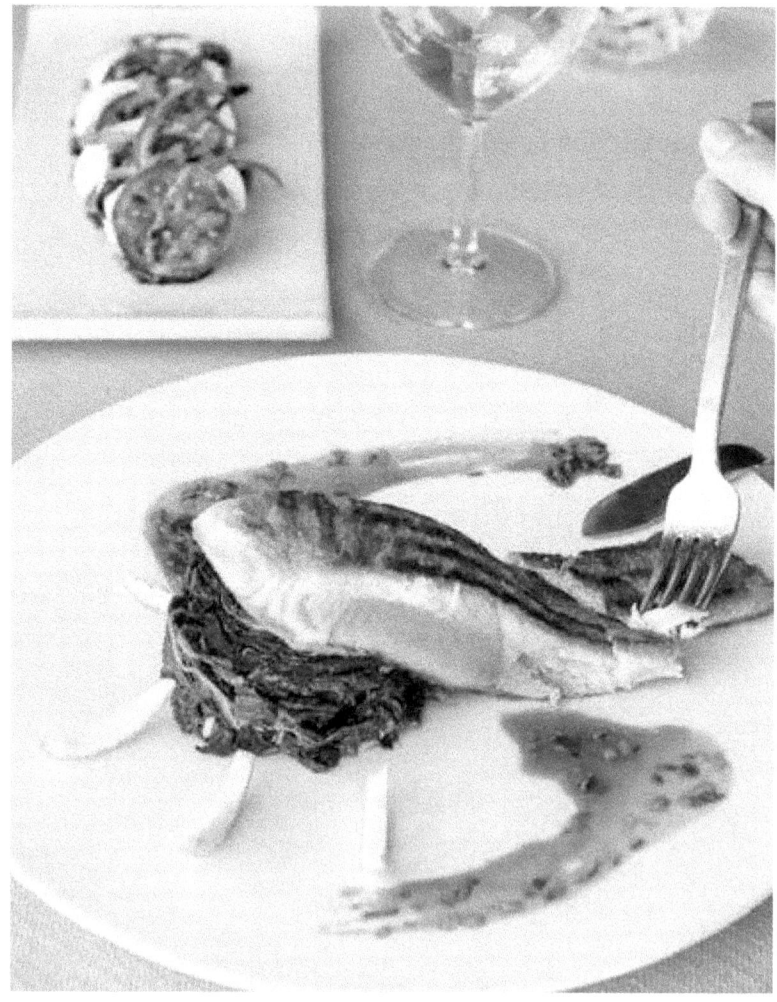

Asian Steamed Fish

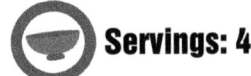 **Servings: 4**   **Cooking Time: 1 hour**

Ingredients:

- 2 tablespoons sugar
- 4 salmon fillets, boneless
- 2 tablespoons soy sauce
- ¼ cup olive oil
- ¼ cup veggie stock
- 1 small ginger piece, grated
- 6 garlic cloves, minced
- 2 tablespoons Worcestershire sauce
- 1 bunch leeks, chopped
- 1 bunch cilantro, chopped

Directions:

1. Put the oil in your Crock Pot, add leeks and top with the fish.
2. In a bowl, mix stock with ginger, sugar, garlic, cilantro and soy sauce, stir, add this over fish, cover and cook on High for 1 hour.
3. Divide fish between plates and serve with the sauce drizzled on top.

Asian Salmon Mix

 **Servings: 2**   **Cooking Time: 3 hours**

Ingredients:

- 2 medium salmon fillets, boneless
- Salt and black pepper to the taste
- 2 tablespoons soy sauce
- 2 tablespoons maple syrup
- 16 ounces mixed broccoli and cauliflower florets
- 2 tablespoons lemon juice
- 1 teaspoon sesame seeds

Directions:

1. Put the cauliflower and broccoli florets in your Crock Pot and top with salmon fillets.
2. In a bowl, mix maple syrup with soy sauce and lemon juice, whisk well, pour this over salmon fillets, season with salt, pepper, sprinkle sesame seeds on top and cook on Low for 3 hours.
3. Divide everything between plates and serve.

Arugula and Clams Salad

 **Servings: 4**   **Cooking Time: 1 hour**

Ingredients:

- 1 cup clams
- 1 cup of water
- 1 garlic clove, diced
- 2 cups arugula, chopped
- 1 tablespoon lemon juice
- 1 tablespoon olive oil

Directions:

1. Pour water in the Crock Pot.
2. Add clams and close the lid.
3. Cook the clams on High for 1 hour.
4. Then drain water and put the clams in the salad bowl.
5. Add arugula and garlic.
6. After this, sprinkle the salad with olive oil and lemon juice and carefully mix.

Basil-Parmesan Shrimps

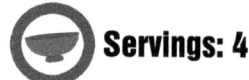 **Servings: 4**   **Cooking Time: 3 hours**

Ingredients:

- 1 tablespoon grass-fed butter, melted
- 1-pound shrimps, shelled and deveined
- 2 cloves of garlic, minced
- 2 tablespoons lemon juice, freshly squeezed
- 1 cup grass-fed heavy cream
- ½ cup fresh basil leaves, chopped
- Salt and pepper to taste
- 1 cup organic parmesan cheese, grated

Directions:

1. Place butter in the CrockPot. Add in the shrimps, garlic, and lemon juice on top. Mix until combined.
2. Stir in the cream and basil leaves. Season with salt and pepper to taste.
3. Sprinkle parmesan cheese on top.
4. Close the lid and cook on high for 2 hours or on low for 3 hours.

Apricot and Halibut Saute

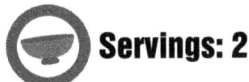 **Servings: 2**   **Cooking Time: 5 hours**

Ingredients:

- 6 oz halibut fillet, chopped
- ½ cup apricots, pitted, chopped
- ½ cup of water
- 1 tablespoon soy sauce
- 1 teaspoon ground cumin

Directions:

1. Put all ingredients in the Crock Pot.
2. Close the lid and cook the fish sauté on Low for 5 hours.

Apple Cider Vinegar Sardines

 Servings: 4   **Cooking Time: 4.5 hours**

Ingredients:

- 14 oz sardines
- 1 tablespoon butter
- ¼ cup apple cider vinegar
- ½ teaspoon cayenne pepper
- 4 tablespoons coconut cream

Directions:

1. Put sardines in the Crock Pot.
2. Add butter, apple cider vinegar, cayenne pepper, and coconut cream.
3. Close the lid and cook the meal on Low for 4.5 hours.

Almond Shrimp and Cabbage

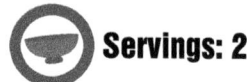 Servings: 2   Cooking Time: 1 hour

Ingredients:

- 1 pound shrimp, peeled and deveined
- 1 cup red cabbage, shredded
- 1 tablespoon almonds, chopped
- 1 cup cherry tomatoes, halved
- 1 tablespoon balsamic vinegar
- 2 tablespoons olive oil
- ½ cup tomato passata
- A pinch of salt and black pepper

Directions:

1. In your Crock Pot, mix the shrimp with the cabbage, almonds and the other ingredients, toss, put the lid on and cook on High for 1 hour.
2. Divide everything into bowls and serve.

Alaska Salmon with Pecan Crunch Coating

 **Servings: 6**   **Cooking Time: 6 hours 30 minutes**

Ingredients:

- ½ cup fresh bread crumbs
- ½ cup pecans, finely chopped
- 6 lemon wedges
- Salt and black pepper, to taste
- 3 tablespoons butter, melted
- 3 tablespoons Dijon mustard
- 5 teaspoons honey
- 6 (4 ounce) salmon fillets
- 3 teaspoons fresh parsley, chopped

Directions:

1. Season the salmon fillets with salt and black pepper and transfer into the crock pot.
2. Combine honey, mustard and butter in a small bowl.
3. Mix together the parsley, pecans and bread crumbs in another bowl.
4. Brush the salmon fillets with honey mixture and top with parsley mixture.
5. Cover and cook for about 6 hours on LOW.
6. Garnish with lemon wedges and dish out to serve warm.

BBQ Shrimps

 **Servings: 6**   **Cooking Time: 40 minutes**

Ingredients:

- 1/3 cup BBQ sauce
- ¼ cup plain yogurt
- 1-pound shrimps, peeled
- 1 tablespoon butter

Directions:

1. Melt butter and mix it with shrimps.
2. Put the mixture in the Crock Pot.
3. Add plain yogurt and BBQ sauce.
4. Close the lid and cook the meal on High for 40 minutes.

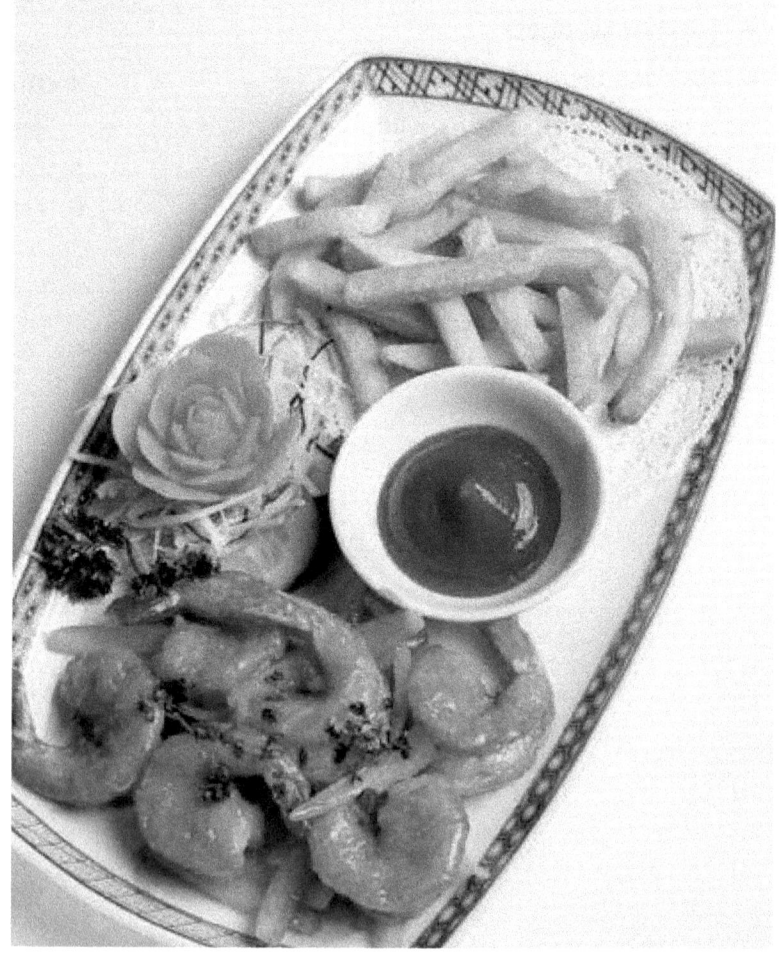

Bigeye Jack Saute

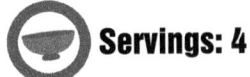 **Servings: 4**   **Cooking Time: 6 hours**

Ingredients:

- 7 oz (bigeye jack) tuna fillet, chopped
- 1 cup tomato, chopped
- 1 teaspoon ground black pepper
- 1 jalapeno pepper, chopped
- ½ cup chicken stock

Directions:

1. Put all ingredients in the Crock Pot and close the lid.
2. Cook the saute on Low for 6 hours.

Braised Lobster

 Servings: 4   **Cooking Time: 3 hours**

Ingredients:

- 2-pound lobster, cleaned
- 1 cup of water
- 1 teaspoon Italian seasonings

Directions:

1. Put all ingredients in the Crock Pot.
2. Close the lid and cook the lobster in High for 3 hours.
3. Remove the lobster from the Crock Pot and cool it till room temperature

9 781804 461235